IT'S IN THE BAG
AND
UNDER
THE
COVERS

Stories of Dating, Intimacy, Sex, & Caregiving
About People with Ostomies

BRENDA ELSAGHER

IT'S IN THE BAG
AND
UNDER
THE
COVERS

Stories of Dating, Intimacy, Sex, & Caregiving
About People with Ostomies

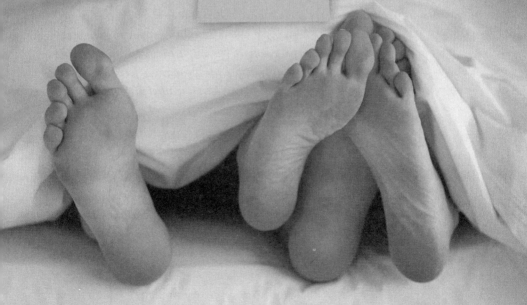

BRENDA ELSAGHER

PRAISE FOR *It's in the Bag and Under the Covers*

A groundbreaking book that openly and honestly addresses sexual intimacy with an ostomy. Brenda compiles real-life stories from real people who have turned the end into a new beginning.

—Mark Vande Kerkhoff, Regional Vice President Managed Care,
Byram Healthcare

This book offers vicarious views of a usually taboo subject. With stories ranging from heart-warming to shockingly unimaginable, it provides an education of life that is unattainable in a classroom.

—Joy Hooper, RN, CWOCN, Anatomical Aprons by Joy

Thank you for writing this book; it reminds me that despite the outer packaging of our bodies, we are the same inside. We all have the desire to get the most out of life and handle the bumps along the way. Life is always worth it.

—Julie Scott, St. Luke's Hospital, Boise, ID

Wow! The stories took me on an emotional roller coaster ride! I found myself laughing, gasping, grieving, and having a strong desire to comfort the ostomate. These stories are affirmations for any ostomate and/or partner with an appliance questioning the possibility of a physical relationship. I can easily foresee this book being recommended pre- and post-operatively by gastrointestinal surgeons who care about the holistic recovery of their patients!

—Lori Hayden, RN, Ostomy Support Group Facilitator,
Carolinas Medical Center-NorthEast, Concord, NC

Sharing heals and these intimate stories provide recovery not only to the story-teller, but also to the receiver of the telling! Living life to the hilt is an absolute universal desire and surviving, also is a collective goal. These stories hit the target and then some as they meet these goals with clarity, humor, direction, purpose, and good intentions. Let the healing begin.

—Erika Hanson Brown, Mayor Pro-Tem of ColonTown

I loved this book. There is such warmth to each interaction, and I believe it will be a positive contribution to people with ostomies.

—Carolyn Hendrix, RN, MSNc, OCN, Director of Oncology,
Hoag Hospital

This book will benefit our patient population at Henrico Doctors' Hospital, as these stories are relative, will keep people engaged, and give helpful advice along the way.

—Brenda Woodcock, RN, MS, WHNP, Administrative Director,
Oncology Services, Henrico Doctor's Hospital

While reading these touching stories, it feels like reality TV inside a book. You are glimpsing into the private, intimate experiences of ostomates and their loved ones as they not only share but reassure that life does go on albeit several adjustments, mishaps, new coping skills, and attitude changes. These sincere authors of all ages, genders, nationalities, do candidly and unabashedly tune in to the most important point that having a pouch does not mean the end of the world.

As a WOC Nurse, I learned plenty that I will pass on to both preoperative and postoperative ostomates who are scared to ask about the intimacy topic. This book will be on our hospital library shelf because sometimes this topic is taboo, hush hush for folks who won't discuss it with the provider. Since the ostomate or caregiver may not ask the pertinent sexual-related questions, it will be there for the taking. The reader can allay his/her anxieties and especially learn that he/she is not alone with fears about dating, marriage, and much more. Thank you, Brenda, for compiling these true, personal stories to create an enlightening book.

—Nancy Scott, RN, BSN, CWOCN, Moffitt Cancer Center,
Tampa, Florida

Quotations from Miss Manners and Robert Sternberg used with permission.

ISBN 978-1-936953-13-4

Library of Congress Catalog Number: 2011929075

Printed in the United States of America
First Printing: May 2011
15 14 13 12 11 5 4 3 2 1

Andover, Minnesota

Expert Publishing, Inc.
14314 Thrush Street NW,
Andover, MN 55304-3330
1-877-755-4966
www.expertpublishinginc.com

——— ✿ ———

OTHER BOOKS BY BRENDA ELSAGHER

If the Battle is Over, Why Am I Still in Uniform?

I'd Like to Buy a Bowel Please!

Bedpan Banter

—— ☙ ——

DEDICATION

For all caregivers—your love, patience, and kindnesses shown in a million small ways will not be forgotten and we are thankful.

For my mother—you taught us how to care for others, and then graciously allowed us to care for you.

And for the person struggling right now to find their way to good physical or mental health as they deal with their ostomy, may you find the daily strength and support you need with a touch of courage, peace, and humor along the way.

CONTENTS

FOREWORD

I chose to practice medicine because I have always been a natural helper. I chose to specialize in Obstetrics and Gynecology because I have always been a family man, and I wanted to help others have healthy sexual lives and be able to establish families as they desired. I developed an interest in cancer care because it seemed to me particularly tragic when a disease that threatens life itself would also threaten fertility and sexual function, human capabilities that lie at the very center of who we are as people.

When I met Brenda in October 1995, this thirty-nine-year-old mother of two small children had been found to have rectal cancer. She had a tumor in the lower anterior wall of the rectum, which would require removal of the anus along with the rectum and lower colon for surgical cure. She would require a colostomy to maintain bowel function.

To obtain adequate margins of normal tissue around the cancer, it would be necessary to remove the posterior wall of the vagina along with the uterus in order to perform this deep pelvic operation. The resulting gaping defect in the perineal area would be difficult to close, and it would be an even greater challenge to preserve her capacity for sexual relations.

Brenda had enjoyed a healthy sexual relationship with her husband, Bahgat, and she expressed concern about strain upon her marriage if she were to be unable to have sexual relations. Her surgeon referred her to me requesting that I assist him with the reconstruction to preserve her sexual function. He knew I had a special interest in gynecological cancer surgery, and I had performed reconstructive procedures for other patients.

Surgical treatment of cancer has often been associated with disfigurement or loss of some bodily function and dread of that outcome has led patients in some cases to avoid treatment. Our ability to perform a reconstructive procedure may lessen the impact of cancer surgery, and markedly enhance the quality of life for one living with the diagnosis of cancer. Great strides have been made in the development of reconstructive procedures, such as the creation of a neovagina, or a neobladder and continent urostomy.

Given my interest in preservation of healthy sexual function wherever possible, my surgical practice has increasingly involved reparative or reconstructive procedures. This complex surgery involves the visualization of a tissue flap, which is shaped to conform to the surgical defect being repaired. It is essential to maintain blood supply to the graft in order to maintain viability and favor healing, and imperative that one be able to close the site from which the graft is taken.

Vulvar skin is elastic, richly supplied with blood vessels, and is close to the vaginal area, so it may be used to reconstruct the vagina. It will, however, continue to grow hair in the new internal location, and this may be a concern as the hair must be removed during periodic medical examinations. For most women, a better alternative is creation of a skin flap from the inner thigh, but the defect on the inner thigh is closed under some tension—there may be more pain, and healing may be slower. There are limitations to the outcome if there is underlying disease such as diabetes, obesity, or poor circulation. Fortunately, successful reconstruction is possible for many healthy women.

As Brenda and I discussed her necessary repair, there were many unknowns in terms of healing and scarring, but she was highly motivated to preserve her sexual function. Therefore, I was confident that if problems did occur, we would be able to manage them by dilation or surgical revision if necessary, and I was committed to do my very best.

Brenda was understandably terrified by her diagnosis, but she also was confident in her ability to fight, and she was willing to place her future in our hands with a great deal of trust. I knew the best time to achieve optimal reconstruction is at the time of the original surgery, and success would hinge in large part upon my ability to match the flaps I could create with the defect I must close.

I did not want to betray her trust by coming unprepared to her operation. I spent hours with my anatomy texts reviewing the precise relationships between muscles, blood vessels, and overlying tissues. I analyzed the length of flap that would be possible versus the length that would be necessary to achieve the desired depth of the vagina. I drew on paper the vulvar anatomy, and laid out flaps as I thought I would be able to create them; I practiced the rotation of them and the internal placement so as to be able to reconstruct the vagina. I did the operation so many times in my head that there were very few surprises on the day of surgery.

Everything came together as planned with good depth and diameter, and the external wounds closed nicely. The postoperative healing went well, and Brenda has assured me on many occasions that her sexual capabilities, although not the same as prior to the operation, are adequate enough and she has the good grace in her life to be pleased with those results.

Throughout my professional life my most common prayer has been that God would help me to do my very best, and that my patient would not suffer if there were some defect in my effort to help her. That prayer was answered in Brenda's case.

I am sure that both Brenda and Bahgat had to make adjustments in their expectations for their sex life as they adjusted to the new anatomical realities. She has spoken eloquently on the topic of dealing with colostomy. I am thankful that through our efforts she has become a cancer survivor who does not also need to talk about the loss of her ability to have sexual relations. Brenda has discovered the value of humor in helping her to deal with changes in her life. She has shared her natural wit with many people through her books, and, as a result, she has probably helped thousands of people cope with their ostomies.

Body image is important to all of us, but who we are is much deeper than that. Our bodies will change with illness, injury, and age. We all need to accept those changes with some dignity in order to be happy in this life. The largest sexual organ in the human body is the cerebral cortex. To focus excessively upon the visible sexual organs or upon an ostomy bag is to miss the point entirely. Brenda has shown us that a bit of humor can go a long way to help us deal with adversity in life and love.

—Leslie A. Sharpe, MD, retired OB/GYN Surgeon

—— ✤ ——

PREFACE

Annually, patients are asked to sign a new HIPAA (Health Information Portability and Accountability Act) form that provides patients with the right to release or limit their protected health information. You can also find out to whom your medical information has been released, or file complaints if you have a dispute. The goal of this regulation is to protect your personal information within your health records. HIPAA was enacted by Congress and signed into law by President Clinton on August 21, 1996.

One of the goals of HIPAA was to ensure that health care providers protect electronic records about patients in the same manner that hard copy records are secured. This way the health care industry could improve their services and further security would lead to more implementation of electronic transactions. One reason that HIPAA was enacted was because the U.S. Federal Government wanted all Medicare transactions to occur electronically and before Congress could mandate patient records, the protection and privacy of patient records needed to be guaranteed.

Even though HIPAA was enacted in 1996, the health care companies had a compliance deadline of 2003. Prior to 1996 and until 2003, we had special visitor training programs offered at many of the local ostomy support groups. It was most often taught by our local WOC Nurse (Wound Ostomy Continence Nurse) and focused on how to talk about adjusting to an ostomy, and we were to talk about our own positive experiences with this life-giving surgery.

In our local chapter of the United Ostomy Association, we had someone who kept busy finding volunteers to visit with people who were new to the ostomy world, whether they were permanent or temporary ostomies. Often the nurses would call from the hospitals with permission from the patient to set up a visit. If possible, the volunteer would match the new ostomate with a same sex person living with an ileostomy, colostomy, or urostomy, depending on which operation the new patient had needed.

During those years, I was a volunteer visitor to many people who were new to having an ostomy. I would go to their hospital rooms most of the time and often speak to the patient along with a family member that might be present. It was good for the patient to be able to talk to someone else that had an ostomy and recognize that it wasn't visible through the clothes, that the visitor didn't stink, or what other strange notions we get as we deal with this new scary world of ostomies.

One of the patients got discharged so rapidly I needed to do a home visit. Her husband was there and I recall a conversation that I've had many times with other people who had ostomies in the hospital. "Can we still have sex?" I would usually try to answer in a light manner. "Well, did you enjoy sex with him/her before the operation?" Since I was talking to mainly women, I didn't have to deal with some of the complications that men went through. For some men, the mechanics don't always work quite the same after ostomy surgery, and it can be sad. There are a few stories in this book that will address that.

For women, it was usually more a case of feeling pretty, finding the right apparel to wear that added to the romance. Yes—was the answer, unless you had other medical complications. Will things be different? Maybe a little—it might take time to adjust. Will he/she still love me with a pouch hanging off of me? That is a good question. I have learned from collecting the stories in this book that everyone reacts differently. I wish I could tell you that yes, they will love you even more knowing what you have gone through, but that isn't always the case. I will say that more often than not people that are in committed, healthy relationships experience no difference except for more compassion for one another, including feeling abundant gratitude for the caregivers.

Over the years, this subject has come up at conferences, newsletters, magazine articles, and most recently, the Internet. It seems that is the safest place to talk about sex and ostomies because of the privacy that comes with having an online identity. You will see it often discussed on public forums, on chat lines, and when someone tells a sad story about being dumped by a boyfriend that couldn't handle seeing the ostomy, there are very compassionate and encouraging remarks back to that writer, encouraging them to keep looking for someone more suitable.

It was some time ago when an associate at Hollister Incorporated, Mary Rome, took me aside and told me that very often people are asking about sexuality issues in phone calls at their direct line consumer programs. When the patients get discharged these days, hopefully their WOC Nurse has provided them with a discharge kit that will not only include products they may need, but one or two other ones to try, along with some educational materials. They might encourage them to follow up with the Secure Start Program that Hollister provides. This program helps the new patient figure out how to order their supplies, how to handle insurance questions, and also get answers about other information like product usage or help with finding valuable resources. They also have WOC Nurses on staff to answer more complex issues that need addressing.

Because of the HIPAA law, hospital and home visits are rare. These days many people seek information from online resources. This kind of program that is offered is extremely helpful to the new patient. I wish I had a program like that fifteen years ago; it would have been so helpful to call someone to ask if I was putting on the pouch correctly. Much like learning to drive a car, it feels like there are many steps to remember, but after a short time, it becomes automatic.

Mary shared with me, "Brenda, many people call our help line asking about making love and having concerns that their ostomy may be a turn off to their partners. Others wonder when is the right time to tell people they are dating and what's the best way to go about that? Have you ever thought about writing anything on this subject?"

"As a matter of fact I have," I said and then, thanks to Mary, the idea became firmly planted.

I will give my limited credentials here to say that I am not in the medical field, I am not a psychologist, (although having previously been a hairstylist, people say I could qualify); instead, I am a lover of people and their stories. This book is not meant to be clinical; it has real stories by real, everyday, ordinary kind of people, like you and me. I was not aiming for humor in this book as much as an honest telling of how these regular folks handled dating, intimacy, sex, and caregiving during this time with their ostomies. I wanted an inside scoop so we could understand the tension we may face, or the relief we may find, in knowing we are not alone. Perhaps a new ostomate will gain knowledge on how to handle telling their date about their ostomy, or a reader may realize it will take some time for them or their partner to adjust to their ostomy and that's okay, too. May this book be just the first opening for other stories to be shared.

ACKNOWLEDGMENTS

For the many brave souls that contributed honestly about their trials and tribulations dealing with dating, intimacy, sex, and caregiving, my wish is that your stories will liberate others to know that even though they may have a difficult situation, perhaps with time, they will learn a different way to cope and aim to live in the hope for good days ahead.

To Sharron Stockhausen for the editing work you did in this book; it required a lot and your creative ideas were helpful as usual.

To Chris Dellwo, Shelly Robinson, and Amy Elsen, thanks for your assistance.

To Jay Monroe for the excellent cover design.

To Dr. Leslie Sharpe, whose excellent surgical skills allowed me to have a continued sex life these last fifteen years. Bahgat thanks you, too.

Sue Hetland, a nurse at Fairview Southdale who cared for my very ill father and let me talk one night about this book and the vision I had for it. Three hours later, she came back with the title. I am grateful for your care and your creativity.

To the United Ostomy Associations of America and Canada, board and advisory members, chapters, and various members, thanks for the work you do on behalf of the ostomates and their loved ones in North America. I am amazed and humbled by the time that is given selflessly by the many volunteers that keep these organizations running. You are the beacon of hope in the positive message you give on living well with an ostomy.

Thanks to C3Life.com and MeetAnOstoMate.com. This book was born out of the many stories I received through your online resources, and I thank you for providing an important resource where people with ostomies can connect, get information, comfort, and encourage one another.

To Aileen Gould for providing many information resources.

To Hollister Incorporated, for being the forerunner in daring to let the people with ostomies tell their own stories about dating, intimacy, sexuality, and caregiving with all their struggles and triumphs. Thank you for helping to provide this forum.

For my family and the constant support you give me by leaving me alone to write or bringing me the occasional cup of tea, along with your heartfelt love, understanding, and patience—I'll be making a home-cooked meal again soon.

Many of the stories in this book were possible through the popular social networking sites of C3life.com and MeetAnOstoMate.com. Here are the brief histories of these two helpful online communities.

C3Life.com

C3Life.com is a website dedicated to helping people with ostomies live their lives to the fullest. It was launched in January 2008, and is supported by Hollister Incorporated, a leading manufacturer of ostomy products. C3Life.com is an outgrowth of Hollister's mission to help make life more rewarding and dignified for those who use its products.

The goal of C3Life.com is to provide a valued, online source of relevant information, connections, and support in one place to help people resume and enrich their lives after ostomy surgery. On C3Life.com, visitors can read about a variety of lifestyle topics, including healthy living, family and relationships, travel, and work/life. They can find information on ostomy-related health issues, products, news, and events. C3Life.com also features blogs written by people who know what it's like to live with an ostomy, including one by Brenda Elsagher.

In addition, those who sign up to be a member of the C3Life Community can pose questions through the site's "Ask the Clinician Panel" feature, share their thoughts via an interactive discussion forum, and submit other content, including personal stories, photos, and videos. They also can elect to receive newsletters that give updates on new site content and provide information on new and interesting ostomy-related products and services.

C3Life.com recently celebrated its third birthday and currently has over eight thousand members. For both new and experienced people with ostomies, life after stoma surgery can be challenging. But there's no need to feel alone when someone to talk to is just a few clicks away.

MeetAnOstoMate.com
Julian Markov

I worked for an ostomy supplies company for about seven years and after I left in 2005, I decided it would be a shame not to use my ostomy-related knowledge. I thought about the issues people with ostomy face and thought I should be able to do something to help. My first idea was to create software that would help both new patients and more experienced ones to find the right ostomy products. The idea came from the fact that many patients come out of the hospital with very little knowledge about ostomy and what choices they have in terms of products. Most patients come out of the hospital with a few samples and have no idea there are at least six different ostomy manufacturers with many different product lines to choose from.

Thus, the idea for a software came alive, to compare products between various manufacturers. If you were to use a particular product, after you typed in the product number, the software would show you alternatives from other manufacturers (with product numbers, descriptions, and pictures). The patient could then either call these manufacturers or request samples from their ostomy supplier.

Unfortunately the software did not gain much popularity, although I approached both patients and nurses. I stopped offering the software for download about a year or two ago, since I did not have the time to maintain its huge database.

Shortly after I launched the software, I remembered how many of our customers at the ostomy supplies company complained about challenges they faced in their private lives. Some of these issues were not being able to start a relationship, their current relationship collapsing because of the ostomy, not knowing anyone else with an ostomy to talk to, etc. Then I thought, *Well, there are a lot of people with an ostomy in North America and around the world, why don't I start a dating website?* So I purchased a software script for that purpose and started building it and learning along the way.

I was quite aware that not everyone would like the idea because an ostomy-dating website might be perceived as a statement that people with ostomy could not be in a relationship with someone without an ostomy. This was definitely not the case. My thinking was that if I can reach out to those few who would feel more comfortable sharing their story (and life) with someone who understands, then I would have achieved my goal.

So, MeetAnOstoMate.com was launched. There were challenges and unhappy faces, mostly from the existing well-established organizations, but I also got a lot of help, too. In time, MeetAnOstoMate.com evolved. I added plenty of features and it became more of a social network than a dating website. The forum was blooming, members were giving each other invaluable support, and I had a few nurses that agreed to participate and share their knowledge and experience.

These days MeetAnOstoMate.com has a forum, blogs, chat rooms, private chat, internal private messaging system, photo gallery, store, events section, classifieds, and many other features. The website is not a typical ostomy-related community, but rather a vibrant multi-topic website, where people have fun, discuss various things, laugh together, cry together, and give each other plenty of love.

The strongest feature of the website is the functionality that allows one to search for other people with an ostomy. There are many different types of searches—by location, gender, age, interests, etc. Members use this feature all the time to either find someone to talk to or to even start a relationship. We offer a few success stories on the website, mentioned in the forum or in the blogs.

MeetAnOstoMate.com is one of the greatest (although small in world terms) online communities. The best part is that people in the community care for each other. I am very proud to have achieved such success and to be able to help people in need.

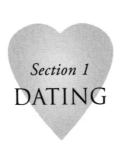

There are three possible parts to a date, of which at least two must be offered: entertainment, food, and affection. It is customary to begin a series of dates with a great deal of entertainment, a moderate amount of food, and the merest suggestion of affection. As the amount of affection increases, the entertainment can be reduced proportionately. When the affection *is* the entertainment, we no longer call it dating. Under no circumstances can the food be omitted.

~Miss Manners' Guide to Excruciatingly Correct Behavior

If we only had Miss Manners to guide us all through the mysteries of dating, it seems like it would be so uncomplicated. Add a dash of humor and some food and I am sure most of us can get through anything. Many people bravely shared their dating escapades in the following stories. You may be a person who is interested in how to tell someone you are dating about your ostomy. I hope you find the answer here.

You will read about the "ostomates" interspersed with "people with ostomies" throughout this book. Both are politically correct in this context as each writer expresses themselves uniquely.

There are some common events that ostomates have that I would bet the average person will not experience. At those tricky, awkward moments, it becomes about attitude and how to deal with surprises in our days—and nights—or our afternoon delights.

Contributors were welcomed to give their stories anonymously if preferred. I tried to get a mix of population, and I happily accepted most of what I received. Most of the stories written were given to me over the phone in interviews, and a few people sent in their own. Most stories went back and forth several times over the last eighteen months and, as lives changed, so did their stories—with rewrites. There are contributors from Europe, Canada, and the USA, thanks to the Internet and the ostomy sites that bring people together.

Dating is different around the world and has certainly changed in the last one hundred years in the USA. In my husband's family in Egypt, there were arranged marriages in the generation before us. These days the young people have input as to whom they wish to marry.

Having six sisters and one brother growing up, people would always tease my dad on the subject of weddings, "How are you going to handle all those girls?" My dad would answer, "I've got some convents lined up or a strong ladder!" Somehow, he's managed just fine.

I grew up with people saying, "It would be good to meet a nice boy in church." That would have never brought my husband and me together since he was raised Muslim in Egypt and I was raised Catholic in Minnesota.

I used to be embarrassed by the way we met each other. Destiny brought us together during the time of the eighties when people had classified ads in newspapers prior to online dating. One night after a couple of adult beverages with a girlfriend, we decided to write the ads and send them in. I could tell one of the people that answered my ad was from another country. I love to travel and get to know people from all over the world, so I agreed to meet him. That night, he brought his brother along and that's how I met my husband.

I am not hung up on how we met anymore; I'm just glad we did. Two children and over twenty-five years of history together, we are still learning from each other and enjoy one another—most of the time!

I did not have an ostomy when we met, so I can only imagine the difficulty some people have in disclosing this to their date. Many people talk about how an ostomy is a great screening device to separate the not-so-swell people from the good people. I didn't have an ostomy, but I was always overweight. That was my own personal screening I suppose, and many people have other kinds of challenges that will weed out the undesirables.

Many stories illustrate that having an ostomy doesn't deter most people from getting to know someone they are interested in. People see past our problems—we all have them, some are visible and some are not.

Perhaps one thing we can learn from these stories is the common thread of once we accept our ostomies, in most cases, other people do too. For those that don't accept our ostomies, it doesn't seem to take long for us to figure out that it's time to move on.

One contributor mentions that if you are excessively worried about being accepted with an ostomy, then either the person isn't right for you or you need to work on self-acceptance. There is much wisdom in the following pages.

————— ✾ —————

YOU CAN DO ANYTHING
AILEEN GOULD

It seems that the words Crohn's, colitis, and ostomy have been a constant in my life. My younger brother was diagnosed with colitis in 1969. Things calmed down for a while but then, with a combination of adolescent hormones and the stress of his bar mitzvah, he had a very bad flare that necessitated ileostomy surgery to save his life. Right after surgery he told our mother he felt his life was over and he would never be able to date or get married.

As he matured, he found a way to explain his situation, started dating, married a beautiful woman, and has two very handsome sons. My other brother went to college and on to medical school, and influenced by our brother, he became a gastroenterologist in 1977.

I was diagnosed with Crohn's disease in 1983 when I was thirty-three years old and divorced.

I told my doctor brother, "No way, no how, are you *ever* giving me a bag on my side!"

He replied, "Aileen, I certainly hope we never have to do that, but there may come a time when the quality of your life is so poor that you will ask us to do it."

"That will never happen," I said.

Eight years later I had no quality of life and realized I had to have a colostomy if I wanted to enjoy my life. I called my brother and said, "I'm ready now."

Fortunately for me, I could also ask my younger brother, who had the ileostomy, some questions. The one I remember most was, "How did you manage it—how did you deal with telling people about it?"

The wisest words I ever heard from him were, "When I accepted it, everyone else accepted it."

Through the years that perspective helped me immeasurably. I went to a general surgeon in 1991 and became the first person ever to have a colostomy done laparoscopically. I was very lucky because I wasn't cut down the middle. A hole was made above my pubic bone and one hole by my belly button—no scars essentially. They put the laparoscopic camera in and looked on a screen to see where they were going without having to cut me open. Once the camera was in, they put a hook in the other hole to make sure they could hook the bowel. If that didn't work, they couldn't do it laparoscopically, but they were able to grab the bowel. Before the surgery, the WOC Nurse had drawn with a magic marker on my stomach where the ostomy was going to be. They then cut that area out and took another hook and pulled the bowel out and laid it on my stomach and cut to form the stoma. Much to the doctors' surprise, my stoma was working immediately and I was out of the hospital in three days.

Shortly after surgery, I met a man who was a chiropractor. Since he was informed about health issues, I told him about my colostomy. We were friends first, got to know each other, had great chemistry, and eventually became sexually intimate. After I had been seeing him for a while and felt secure in the relationship, I asked him, "Does it bother you that I have a bag on my side?"

"Oh, really—where? I didn't notice it," he said.

"Oh, I love you," was my quick reply.

There have been other men since that relationship, and I usually tell the guy on the second or third date that I was sick a while back. If they ask questions, I tell them more about Crohn's disease, and if I feel we are going to be sexually intimate, before we get into the bedroom, I'll remind them of the earlier conversation.

"Remember I told you that I used to be sick? I' m better now because I had surgery called a colostomy that requires a little bag on my side. It's like a big bandage on one side. It's no big deal. It won't get in our way, it won't affect us," and with a big smile on my face, I say, "I promise I can do anything we want to do." That was all they needed to hear.

I minimize my ostomy. I don't go into how it works and how I take care of it.

I used to roll it up and tape it down. I don't need to do that anymore because I wear a black lacy hip-T that I learned about on the ostomy discussion board on the Internet. This holds my bag securely for me and it's discreet.

I leave it on while I sleep, which ensures that in the morning they won't see that my bag may have filled with gas or stool.

Several years later, when I was with a different boyfriend, I asked him, "Does it bother you that I have a bag on my side?"

His response, "Have you seen my ankle? When I was eighteen, I broke it playing ball and it will never look the same."

I said, "What are you talking about? It's not a big deal."

He said, "Exactly, Aileen. Everyone has something wrong—who's perfect?"

In my practice as a licensed mental health counselor, I specialize in counseling people with chronic illnesses, particularly people with ostomies. I always give a free initial mini-session to anyone with an ostomy. We'll talk for twenty to thirty minutes, and if they decide they need further help, we will schedule more sessions.

I have found the subject of intimacy seems to be more important for women than men. But I also see that many men have different issues they need to work through.

Many companies make intimate apparel for women. There are fewer items for men but they can get away with wearing a pair of silk underwear. I feel the most important aspect of intimacy is that as each person accepts the ostomy as part of themselves, their partner will too. When joy and intimacy exist in a relationship, a complete and fulfilling life can return and then even improve life in larger ways.

—— ⊛ ——

INTERNET DATING CAN WORK
Barbara Kupferberg

I have been a widow for over five years and, after ostomy surgery, had given up ever finding any sort of romance. I had a problem with my appliance and the medical professionals were not helping much, so I sent out inquiries on an Internet site.

A lovely, kind person answered me and told me he had been an ostomate for four years and it was a trial-and-error process with learning about appliances. He only wished someone had been there to help him.

That was over two years ago and since then we corresponded through the MeetAnOstoMate.com site, exchanged e-mail addresses, and then phone numbers. Although he does not live near me, we have had several visits back and forth. I enjoy his company; he is a smart, funny, and caring human being.

For a long time he teased me, telling me that my only interest in him was that I was grateful to him for his help. We are having a wonderful time, even though the phone lines are burning up more than the airlines.

My children were hysterical at the thought of me going to visit a strange man in a different state. We had talked for hours on the phone and I felt like we were good friends when he met me at the airport. He gave me a big hug and when I got to the car there was a single, red rose lying on the seat. We went to lunch and continued our conversation as if we had known each other for years. Arriving at his home, he took my bags into the guest room and then I noticed a lovely bouquet of flowers that had a card saying, "Welcome to Texas."

Of course, one of the most comfortable parts to our being together is the fact that we have both been through the same thing and that makes the compatibility even better. He was fortunate to have a complete and successful reversal several months ago and I am thrilled for him. After he recuperated, on his visit to see me in Florida, he brought his big dogs; they behaved perfectly in my home, and I am in love with them.

When we were physical, he tucked his pouch into a belt-like thing, and I never paid any attention to it. I bought some of those crotch-less panties on one of the sites, they were pretty—sexy ones, and we just sort of ignored the fact that we had ostomies; it wasn't even a problem. He still teases me and even though I am very discreet, periodically he will say, "Saw a bit of your bag." And then we laugh.

He'd had previous experiences with other women, none of whom seemed to mind. I had no previous experience but was comfortable with the fact that he cared not a bit that I had an ostomy; I am crazy about him. Where this is going? I can't say, but for now, I am having a blast and he is too.

—— ☙ ——

MAKE DATES AND PLAN AHEAD
DAVID AND CEIL McGEE

DAVID McGEE

One night in January 2004, I got up around 3:00 a.m. for another trip to the bathroom, a common occurrence, but I never made it back to bed. I passed out in the bathroom and fell off the toilet and onto the floor. I didn't hurt myself, but when I came to I didn't have the strength to get up. I hated to awaken my wife, so I guess I fell back to sleep on the floor. The next morning she found me and helped me up.

This incident was basically the last straw. For the entire previous week she had tried to help me eat, all the while saying I should be going to the hospital. Having recently started a new job, I was concerned about not having insurance, so I wasn't willing to go. Later that day, I finally agreed to go, and when we realized I was so weak I couldn't get up off the couch to get in the car, she had to call 9-1-1 for help in getting me to the hospital.

I don't remember anything for the next four days. I was told that at the hospital, they did a CAT (Computerized Axial Tomography) scan, but it didn't show anything.

My wife agreed to let them do exploratory surgery to find the problem. What they found was that a blood clot in my superior mesenteric artery had stopped all blood flow to my intestines. Most of my colon and small intestines had essentially died—they were blue. The doctors informed her they could either suture me back up and I would die in my sleep, or they could remove the intestines. She contacted my parents and together they opted for the removal. I had become so dehydrated that they believe this is what caused the blood clot, although I have been tested and am not prone to clotting.

None of this had anything to do with the ulcerative colitis I had been diagnosed with nineteen years earlier. This latest procedure left me with practically no bowels remaining, and everything I eat or drink goes right through my stomach into an ileostomy pouch. Without enough small intestines to absorb anything, I have trouble even simply taking pills and must grind them to get any benefit from them. Now I just eat for the fun of it, I taste foods just fine, but I retain nothing. The small blessing in all this is I can eat anything I want and not gain weight.

To stay alive and get nourishment, I have to hook up to a three-liter bag of TPN (total parenteral nutrition) every day.

I took TPN 24/7 until I was released from the hospital. Once I came home and learned how to do it myself, eventually I was able to speed up the infusion and reduce the time to nine hours at night while I sleep. This gives me some sense of normalcy during the day.

I was approved for social security disability. Six months later my wife then decided she didn't want to deal with me and my complications any longer.

I moved to South Carolina to be closer to family, and soon realized I didn't want to live the rest of my life alone. But, I had a nagging feeling that my chances were not very good for finding a woman who could love me now.

Another six months passed, I signed up for eHarmony and had lots of matches. After several first dates only over the next few months, the relationships never continued. I quickly learned there was no reason to even mention my medical situation under these fleeting circumstances. I determined that only when both the lady and I mutually agreed we'd like to go out again, would I find a way to tell her, knowing this might be the end of things. It took a couple of years to find the right person. Here's her perspective on how we got together:

Ceil McGee

One of David's eHarmony matches had been with my best friend, who repeatedly kept insisting throughout their entire dinner date that she thought he really should meet her best friend, Ceil.

Within a few days, he called me, then we e-mailed some and soon met for lunch. We had an enjoyable time getting to know each other. He was a great listener, asking just the right questions, and we had a lot in common.

I knew he was in his fifties and I had a question for him, "Why are you retired at such a young age?"

He said, "Can you trust me on that point, and I'll get back with you later on that?"

I thought that was a bit odd, but hey, it was only lunch and I was enjoying his company. When I thought more about it, I came to three possible options. One, he had won the lottery but wanted to be sure I was interested in *him*, and not his money. I could live with that. Two, he'd worked in retail and warehouse management for over twenty-five years, so I thought maybe he'd gotten into legal trouble, but I didn't notice any electronic jewelry and he seemed too sincere. Third, perhaps some kind of medical condition, but he certainly seemed healthy, thoughtful, and kind.

We both wanted to see each other again, and David asked if he could stop by my office before we went out the second time. I agreed.

When he arrived he said, "I want to talk with you a little and answer your question about my early retirement." He proceeded to tell me about his twenty years of intestinal illness that had culminated in life-saving surgery with the result of him having an ostomy. He further explained, "I now have to be on IV nutrition for nine to ten hours daily. I am in generally good health otherwise. Things are under control and I manage my medical needs pretty well." Then he offered, "If you don't want to go forward into a relationship, I will understand."

I thought, *well, at this age, anyone can suddenly have health issues, and so okay, major adventures like rock-climbing or sky-diving might not be possible, but they really weren't on my bucket list anyway.* I said, "I don't see it as a hindrance to getting to know each other better."

Next he took me by surprise when he asked, "Have you ever seen an ostomy bag?"

"No" I said.

"Would you like to?" he asked.

"Okay," I said.

When he started to unzip and reach into his pants, I thought, *Whoa, what am I going to see? What have I agreed to?* Of course, it was fine and not gross at all.

We married six months later, and I have been blessed for nearly four years by David's kindness, attention, and love.

We've had some interesting adventures to the emergency room. The first one was only two months after we married, with David passed out cold from accidentally putting too much insulin into his TPN bag. I learned the importance of having all of his medical information, his doctors, medications, etc. written on a card, as I only knew his birth date and social security number. He had always taken care of all of his medical needs prior. I never wanted to answer "I don't know" again and not be his medical advocate.

Even though by nature I'm a bit squeamish, it has never bothered me to change David's IV dressing or occasionally help with an ostomy pouch change. When I look at David, I see a wonderful man, and I see the marvels of medicine that have given us both another chance at love.

I'll add that neither his ostomy nor his TPN nightly infusions have impeded nor interfered with the more intimate aspects of our marriage. We do make dates and plan ahead for those times, and he'll be the first to admit that spontaneity has had to take a back seat now because he must take his ostomy into consideration.

Who knows what adventures we'll experience next, but with faith, love, and a sense of humor, we'll share the rest of our lives together.

—— ⊛ ——

YES, I CAN!
LISA MAYFIELD

I was married when I had ileostomy surgery at age twenty-one. At the time I didn't realize that being married hadn't stopped my husband from dating. After six surgeries for Crohn's disease, I was finally well enough to get on with my life. I discovered my marriage was over when we went out after my surgery with a bunch of people, and I had an accident with my ostomy. My husband had described a friend as a short, fat, dumpy girl but in fact she was the opposite. She was present at the club where I had my accident. That showed me that some things he had been saying weren't true.

I went home to change, while he stayed there. I decided to look for his wedding ring that he hadn't been wearing. When I found it, I found some phone numbers.

On the way back, I was pulled over for speeding and talked my way out of that ticket by saying, "I have a medical issue and I am on my way home to change my ostomy." I lied. The officer gave me the ticket anyway, and when I repeated my story to the judge, I lied in court, too. The judge let me go.

That was in my youth and I would neither condone nor encourage this behavior these days. My husband was in the military; I needed his insurance and he got extra pay for being married. From that night on, we started doing our own thing. Over time, I started getting out in the dating world.

Eventually I met the guy I am married to now. He was a good old red-neck country boy. When it came time to tell him, we were in a restaurant, his favorite—any buffet; he'll eat anything that doesn't eat him first.

"I have something important to tell you and it's kind of serious," I said.

"Right now?" he said, anxious to eat.

"Yes. I have Crohn's disease; I have had surgery for it. After I got done with all the surgery, I've been healthy ever since. This is the deal; they took out the colon, and I have to wear the pouch. Do you understand what I am saying to you?"

He nodded.

"Do you have any questions?" I asked.

He hesitated, "Can you have sex?"

I replied, "Yes, I can."

He continued, "Can you have kids?"

"Yes, I can," I repeated.

"Can we eat now?" he asked as he eyed the buffet.

That was the specifics and that's all he needed then. In time, I taught him how to change the pouch relating it to changing a valve cover gasket. "When you change the valve cover gasket, you have to clean the surface, the metal. You clean off the old one with lacquer thinner, then you put down some glue, some adhesive, and then you put down the valve cover back on top. So you see it's like changing a pouch, you use skin prep or paste your Eakin seal, wafer, and then the pouch." He got it.

I was always comforted by something that Ken Aukett, past president of the United Ostomy Associations of America (UOAA), said once when he gave a talk to a group of us in the 20/40 group from UOAA. He said, "If you're naked, the man's not going to care if you have a pouch." I believed him and have been okay with my pouch when it came to intimate moments.

My husband is nonchalant. My having a pouch doesn't bother him in the least and we have been married nineteen years. Our son is eighteen years old now and he doesn't know me any different. He thought all mommies had ostomies. At first he thought only women had them, not men. He goes to the national convention with me and it's made him more of a compassionate kid. If I had stayed sick, I wouldn't have been able to have him. I work full-time and am a soccer coach with twenty-seven seasons behind me, two seasons a year. I am active, even going to church camp in a room with seventeen people and most people didn't know I had an ostomy. Because I had surgery, I was able to have Devin because I wasn't sick any longer. I went to many national conventions, made many good friends, and my life is better because of the surgery.

—— ☙ ——

DATING PLEASURE
ESTEN GOSE

I am twenty-eight years old and live in Seattle, Washington. I have had my ileostomy for six years now due to my diagnosis of FAP (Familial Adenomatous Polyposis). I was diagnosed at age ten, after my doctors noticed a tumor on my right jaw bone and removed it to be biopsied.

After I was diagnosed, I had a colonoscopy and endoscopy every year or six months, depending on what the previous scope's results were. I had my last colonoscopy six-and-a-half years ago, after which my gastroenterologist informed my parents and me that it was time to remove my entire colon, or I would have stage IV colon cancer within two years.

I realize now that it was the best decision of my life, having my entire colon removed. My surgery was done laparoscopically at the Cleveland Clinic, and after severe life-threatening peritonitis, some major complications, and nine months of healing, I was given an ileostomy at age twenty-two.

After my surgery, I wondered if there would ever be a girl out there who would accept my ostomy. I decided to take a chance, and asked a friend of mine if she had any friends she could set me up with. She said she did have a friend who was single, and she set me up with her. Her friend and I hung out a few times in the beginning, to just kind of feel each other out and see if there was anything there. Hanging out with her became us walking on the beach together, and shortly after that we decided to be together.

From the time we first met, until we started dating, I tried the best I could to hide my ostomy, fearing a bad reaction and that she would not want to hang out around me. Once we started dating, I still wasn't sure I was ready to tell her about my ostomy, and continued to hide it. That plan worked until one day we were in my room watching a movie together, lying on my bed holding each other, and relaxing in each other's comfort.

My stoma, appropriately named "Butthead," decided it wasn't going to let me hide it anymore, and began farting. There was enough air moving out of the stoma that I could not hide it, and so my girlfriend heard it. I looked at her and said to her, "There is something I need to tell you about, and I hope you're okay with it."

I brought her to my computer and told her I have a medical condition that required that my colon be removed, or I would have had colon cancer. I then told her I have what is called an ostomy and explained that it is a pouch attached to my abdomen, where a small portion of my intestines are pulled out to collect my waste. I asked her if she had any questions or concerns. To my surprise, she told me that she was okay with it, and that she liked me for who I was, and that my medical condition would not change that. I was ecstatic to hear her say that as I didn't expect it.

She was really good about accepting my ostomy and over time knew when I needed help or when I needed to use the bathroom or change my pouch. When we would be hanging out with friends, she would keep an eye on me, and if she could tell something was wrong, would ask me about it and if I needed her help with anything. Her support meant everything to me, and I was impressed with the initiative she took when it came to helping care for me.

At one point, as we were watching a movie at home, I felt that burning sensation that tells you it is time to change your pouch. I paused the movie and told her I would be right back, and I was going to change my pouch. She looked at me and asked me if she could come watch me change it because she wanted to see how I did it in case she needed to help me. She watched in amazement as I took the old pouch off, prepped my skin, and put the new wafer and pouch on.

The relationship got to the point where everything was going really well, and our sex life began. Our first time, I asked her if she wanted me to hide my pouch, or use one of the wraps I had to keep the pouch out of the way. She politely told me no, that it wasn't in the way. Each time we had sex, it seemed to get better and better, and it was clear to me that my ostomy was indeed not in the way.

She was the first girl I dated after having my ostomy surgery, and we ended up dating for almost two years. She ended up leaving me one day, waiting until I fell asleep and then she got out of bed, packed all her things, and arranged for a friend to come pick her up. I never heard from her or saw her again. It was very difficult, and I still have no clue why she left me, but I am grateful for the two years I dated her. Even though things didn't turn out for us, she helped me so much in gaining confidence, and showed me that if a girl cares for you enough, she won't let your ostomy or diversion stand in the way.

———— ⊛ ————

BE HONEST AND COURTEOUS
GEORGA A. LINKOUS-LONG

I like to joke that I am an expert at marriage—I've been married four times. My first fiancé I dated fresh out of high school. I didn't have an ileostomy yet but I had a pull-through, where they removed my colon and connected the small intestine to the rectum.

I was a virgin and wanted to save myself until I got married. I met this young man of twenty-three when I was working on Wilmington Island, Georgia, as a waitress. He was the first man that asked me out, and I fell in love at age eighteen. About six months into dating and being his girlfriend, I felt comfortable to lose my virginity at age nineteen. It was that typical awkward, teenager moment and would have been weird regardless of surgery. Not realizing all that had been reconstructed in that area, I wasn't sure if I felt good or bad. I didn't know what I should be feeling and didn't know how to physically respond. I wasn't sure what normal was.

Through more times of having sex, we figured out our own pattern. Later on, the rectal muscles from the surgery were not strong enough to hold back my watery bowel movements, and I ended up having accidents on him. Later, at night, I had to wear diapers and our relationship became more difficult.

I finally had enough and got tired of being sick, so I asked the doctor for an ostomy. I wanted a life. My fiancé's mother took me to have my surgery at Emory University in Atlanta, Georgia.

I didn't realize my fiancé was all about how I looked on the outside. His and my relationship was never the same. He was not attracted to me anymore, and we ended up breaking up. He couldn't support me emotionally. I realized that he would rather have me suffering the way I was living, than to love me with a pouch, so I broke up with him.

Years later, a friend told me my old fiancé was diagnosed with cancer. We reunited by phone and talked about that time in our lives. He apologized for his lack of understanding and told me he was proud of me for moving on and not letting the ostomy get in the way. He used the knowledge he gleaned from me to fight the seven types of cancer he battled but sadly, we lost him recently at only forty-seven years old. Jon Foster's memory lives in our hearts.

In another incident, my dad was in my shop loading up supplies to be delivered when a new customer came in. During the conversation the customer asked me what I could *not* do as an ostomate. I told him, "When I was twenty-one, I ran into a guy from high school days and invited him over to my parents' house to go swimming in their indoor pool while they were out of town. I showed him my ostomy. I had nothing on but a pouch cover and it didn't faze him. There was a Jacuzzi connected to the pool and while skinny dipping, the jet pulled the pouch off and it was floating across and into the pool. He jumped out of the Jacuzzi, got cleaned up, and said, 'I adore you, but I have to go home.' We stayed friends for a long time."

My father's face was blood red, "So you mean to tell me I had to clean that whole damn swimming pool because of a boyfriend?"

I looked at the customer and said, "Fifteen years later and I guess I'm caught now."

My current husband and I met online. I didn't have time to get out and date. I decided to try out the site nocheatersdate.com. My profile said, "I am an ostomate of twenty-five years. I have an ileostomy with multiple health problems. If you don't know what it is, look it up, and if you don't want to deal with me, don't e-mail me."

The first night I had eighty-nine e-mails from both men and women asking me how I dated with an ostomy. I had four marriage proposals. My husband was the only one that went to the website, looked it up, and learned about it.

Overall, when it came to dating, I found out about the person in casual conversation. Basic things like the weather or I might ask questions about them specifically. In most cases I would be upfront about having an ostomy. If I told them later after they had gotten to know me, it was more difficult.

I asked my prospective husband if I could meet him, and he drove seventy miles to see me at my work, then we met half-way for our first date and have continued to meet half-way on many levels. That's when I found out that people needed that honesty, better to get the information out right away to wipe any doubts or fears away.

I found out that being candid and using humor works best, even in the work situation. My coworkers know that if I say, "I have a flat tire," I can instantly become a bio hazard. It's my code for I need to use the bathroom immediately. I try to respect everyone and request the same from them.

I teach ostomy etiquette. For people that have an ostomy, you don't have the right to offend others; you can use spray deodorizer in the room or ostomy appliance deodorant. I teach people how to muffle the sounds to avoid embarrassment. I educate employers on how to handle an employee who has an ostomy to make sure they are not milking the clock. I teach people to wrap their pouches in plastic so the pouches are not exposed in a trash can. Dealing with an ostomy is no reason to not be as courteous as possible.

I could not get through life so well without the friends I have met through my business, outside of work, and even on the social pages on the Internet. It's important for me to be able to joke and be honest with my loved ones. I think being able to laugh about our day-to-day struggles with an ostomy is crucial to our survival, and I'm thankful I can do that.

—— ⊛ ——

TRY BEING ME ONE DAY
Holly St. Jean

When I almost died, everyone was happy. Naturally, I was the happiest. It's a shame when a person *almost* makes the grade, scores the win, or wins the lottery. But, when a person *almost* dies, it's time for celebration. After I *almost* died, I mean, after it sunk in that if not for a skilled surgeon and a team of doctors I would have died, I was euphoric. Things like showering without assistance, eating solid foods, laughing, walking, driving, admiring the beauty of nature filled me with wonder. I spent an entire September day collecting red and yellow Massachusetts maple leaves to send to my friend Kathleen, a freshman attending college in upstate New York. The fact that New York maple leaves were possibly just as beautiful as leaves from home meant little to me; Kathleen would appreciate the gesture. The fact that I was missing my first semester of college to recuperate, well, I *almost* died, but didn't—so no complaining.

Life was great for a while, but then came panic. I'd promised God I'd be ever grateful for this second chance and deal with my new circumstance in a positive way, always. By October, this pledge began gnawing at my gut. Ironic, really, since ulcers had almost killed me in the first place.

Ulcerative colitis, a disease I never knew I had until I collapsed in July, had ravaged my large intestine. And so the intestine and the disease had been removed. Thank goodness for my ileum, the back-up small intestine that would handle things through re-routed plumbing.

Sure, now I wore an appliance, and was referred to as an ileostomate (which sounded like an *Italian pirate*), but I was no longer sick. And being well meant it was time to be the best person I could be. A deal with God was a deal with God.

Even the stunning young woman sent by the ostomy society assured me of this fact. She, too, an "Italian pirate," flashed a photo of herself in a bathing suit, and another of her and her boyfriend dressed in formal wear. Momentarily, she did give me hope, but having only ever been *almost* pretty, rather than envisioning myself with a handsome someone, I saw myself alone, a placard that said, "Unlovable," swinging from my neck. Who would ever want *me*?

Following this young woman's visit, I withdrew. My friends were all off at college, and I was stuck. The thing weighing upon my mind was the fact that I was destined to be a virgin forever. Why had I wasted my time in school strictly worrying about *making* the honor roll instead of *making it* with anyone at least once? I felt like phoning those bad girls in my senior class and congratulating them for knowing how to truly live.

Once I got into college, I dated. I studied, too—art and literature—a double major. Besides trying to make the grades, I made the guys. I also learned my ileostomy was never an issue; the physical experience, not me, was the most important thing for them, and it wasn't enough. I felt like calling those bad girls back and asking, "So, that's it? What's so great about sex? And when does the love kick-in?"

Ten years after college, following an eight-year marriage to a wonderful man, with two years of therapy I secretly attended during the last two years of the marriage, I finally discovered the truth and it was simple: I was gay, and the fact was I really hadn't found the right kind of love yet.

The hardest thing I've ever had to do was tell my husband. Bob asked if I'd ever been unfaithful. He was relieved when I told him no. When I told him I didn't even know another gay person and that the word lesbian frightened me, he wanted to know how I could be sure. "I just am," I said, and that's when we both started to cry.

Since Bob was leaving on a business trip that very evening, I explained that I was leaving too and wouldn't be back when he returned in a few days. There was the moving van, which moved me fifteen miles away to my mother's for a month, then the move to my new apartment, and the move to the courthouse three months later to sign the divorce papers before a judge, and finally, the move to meet my people. Only, where would I find them?

Bob remarried a year after our divorce. He has the two children he always wanted. Several years ago, Bob and I bumped into one another at Home Depot, or as I affectionately refer to it now, Homo Depot. He'd heard that I had bought a house, and that I had a partner. I said I'd heard he'd had a second child. It was a little awkward, but we got through it and the encounter ended with a hug. I picked up the cans of paint I needed for our upstairs bathroom and left the store knowing I'd made the right decision.

Ironically, on the day the movers were loading furniture on the van and as my neighbor and friend Gayle and I were saying our good-byes, she gave me her brother Joey's phone number and told me to call him. Joey was gay and he belonged to a gay and lesbian cultural awareness group in Worcester, Massachusetts, and I went with him to a meeting. I met people, women, and they were kind, intelligent, funny, and human. Eventually, I had a network of new friends and, in time, a couple of romances. I was happy and even discovered a gay and lesbian ostomy group.

These days I am a high school teacher and have lived with my ileostomy for twenty-eight years. I've been in a loving relationship for eleven years. I met Helena at a women's dance when I was thirty-four. A women's dance is an underground, speakeasy kind of thing, locally run, and usually held in a rented Knights of Columbus sort of hall. I'd gone to a couple and enjoyed the music and dancing. And the atmosphere was interesting.

In this world, as in any group, there are differences. I have friends who are both butch and femme. I consider myself to be feminine, and I am attracted to feminine women. That night, there in a sea of butches, was one striking woman who stood out. I noticed her the minute I came in and sat with my friends. She was out there dancing by herself courageously and didn't seem inhibited at all. She was thin and had long dark hair. She wore black pants and a black-and-white, checked blouse. Her arms were lifted over her head for much of the song as she clapped to the beat like a proud flamenco dancer. The song was the new Enrique Iglesias hit "Bailamos."

We all wanted to know who she was; no one had ever seen her. As the song ended, as if in a trance, I uncharacteristically went over to ask her to dance. My friends seemed shocked, and they watched as she shot me down completely with a smile and a shake of her head. I returned to my table feeling like I'd been punched. I drank my beer and watched her sit out this slow song and talk with her friends. Then, when the next song started, a lively rock number, she came over to me directly, took my hand, and led me to the floor. After that, we spent hours talking by the bar.

She had a lovely thick Spanish accent that made my head swim. The music in the room seemed to fade and all I could hear was Helena's voice. She was from Bogota, Colombia, now a school teacher in Worcester. We exchanged numbers on napkins at the end of the evening, and she said she would call me. I didn't believe her. When she called the next day about 11:00 a.m., I was in the shower. I heard my answering machine recording her voice. I let it.

Still soapy, I shut off the water, wrapped a towel around me, and ran to the phone. I replayed her message at least five times before I returned her call. I had never before felt what I was feeling as I kept pushing that button and dripping on the carpet. I couldn't breathe I felt so happy.

We met that afternoon at the café in a book shop. We ate lunch and talked for more hours. I asked her if she'd like to come over to rake leaves the next day, I had just purchased a home and I had yard work to do. Realizing it wasn't the most interesting invitation the moment it launched from my lips, I figured she'd say no. Come over and help me rake leaves? What sort of person extended such an offer to a beautiful woman? But she smiled and agreed.

The next afternoon, Helena showed up. Together we bagged leaves. It was totally ridiculous, and the most fun I'd had in years. Later, we went in for hot chocolate. I made a fire, and things got intimate, but just kissing. We went out quite a few times and one night at her apartment, things started to progress. As they did I backed away and told her, "We have to stop."

I told her I had a disease that required my entire colon be removed, resulting in a permanent ileostomy. My explanation had been more in depth; I had never been more worried telling anyone else. Helena mattered. While I spoke, she did an astonishing thing; she went over to her book case and took down a medical book and instantly started looking it up. She had studied medical terminology and wanted to know all about it. I think she thought I was interesting as a medical case. She had worked at the University of Massachusetts in the hospital for a while before getting a permanent teaching position.

She understood. "It was okay? Is there any pain? How can I touch you?" she asked. "I want to touch you," she said.

I started to cry. Helena kissed away my tears. During intimacy, I can still get upset about the ileostomy. It can make me feel ugly. My mother is a pretty good seamstress and has always made me appliance covers; the one I wore that night was a velvet leopard skin print. I always wear a pouch cover, and I've even gone so far as to add tiny strips of Velcro. This way I can roll it up and make it as small as possible. I don't want it flopping around. It never bothers Helena.

Not that long ago, I experienced a near disaster at school, a leaky bag in the middle of class. I was able to get coverage for my class and able to change my appliance in the faculty bathroom. No one was the wiser, but I was an emotional mess.

When we got home, Helena said, "Let me try it, I want to know what it feels like." She spent the rest of the day wearing one of my Hollister one-piece bags. We filled it up with pudding and she even practiced emptying it before bed. She wore it all night, showered with it the next morning, refilled it with pudding, and headed off to school. She finally removed it after dinner. Who would do this? How can I not love this woman?

Helena is the love of my life, and we teach at the same high school. We have traveled much of the U.S. and Canada, South America, Mexico, and we are headed to Spain. We do everything together and I am hopeful we always will. Helena has always accepted me—all of me.

—— ⊗ ——

LIFE AFTER DIVORCE
Liz Dennis

Life as I once knew it changed forever when I was diagnosed with stage III rectal cancer. I remember my disappointment when I woke up after my first surgery and realized I had an ileostomy. Even though my surgeon said it would be a temporary inconvenience lasting no more than one year, I wondered if I would end up with a permanent colostomy like my father did thirty years prior. Unfortunately, the follow-up surgery a year later to reverse my ileostomy failed. Indeed I ended up with a permanent colostomy.

But I never imagined that my husband of twenty-two years, the father of my two children, the man who vowed to love me in sickness and health, would reject my body. Instead of kissing my scars and thanking God that my surgery had saved my life, he turned away from me. It was as if my cancer had ruined *his* life. There was little concern for how rectal cancer had compromised *my* quality of life. I felt alone and confused. I hardly knew how to cope with my changed body. When I needed my husband more than ever before, he wasn't around.

At first the rejection was subtle. Later my husband really flipped out. He couldn't stand the fact that I wasn't wearing cute, little, sexy panties anymore—that I had switched to larger underwear. He made derogatory comments about my pants with the elastic waists calling them "old lady clothes."

I preferred loose garments after surgery; they felt more comfortable as I adjusted to my new body. I knew our relationship was in trouble. We sought counseling and talked openly about physical intimacy.

I hardly knew how to take care of my ostomy. I remember standing in front of the sink in my bathroom, looking in the mirror, and saying, "I don't think I can do this." My mother provided the support and encouragement I needed to get through those hard moments. But who was going to help me reestablish a sexual relationship with my life partner if he no longer desired my body?

The counselor suggested we experiment. In reality, we were intimate only once during a three-year period. My husband later admitted the only reason he could make love to me that one time was that he was drunk. My ostomy turned him off. He never wanted to have sex with me again. I was banished from our bedroom. His rejection was hurtful and eventually we divorced.

Just when I thought no one could ever love me again, I reconnected with a high school sweetheart I had kept in touch with over the years. I poured out my heart and soul to him about my divorce process, and he shared his problems, too. We had remained great friends over the years and were a good support for each other.

One time during my marriage separation, he came into town from another state and we got together for a visit. Even though he was involved with someone else, and I felt guarded about my body, we were sexually intimate that evening. Our lovemaking felt natural to me. I trusted him and felt safe. My ostomy wasn't an issue. I forgot all about it until I heard a strange sound.

"What's that?" I asked.

"It's just your ostomy bag; it's no big deal," he said reassuringly.

This encounter helped heal the wounds left behind by my husband. However, I still feel apprehensive and afraid of dating someone I don't know. I am grateful to my high school sweetheart for giving me hope. Even though we are not together, he helped me understand that it is possible to love again. I am not my body. I am whole, complete, and loveable.

——— ❦ ———

MY NEW LIFE
MICHAEL HASSETT

In 1982, I unwillingly lost forty pounds from my one-hundred-fifty-pound frame. Over the next twenty-five-year period, what started as irritable bowel syndrome (IBS), progressed to inflammatory bowel disease (IBD), then colitis—eventually became ulcerative colitis. In truth, I had become a prisoner of my bowels *and* the bathroom. Throughout my medical journey, my marriage was falling apart. With a sense of urgency happening each minute, intimacy was gone; trying to consummate the act was impossible. Ten years without intercourse, and masturbated only twice!—not!—but it was time to do something.

I tried the J-pouch route to avoid becoming an ostomate. Completely afraid of ostomy surgery, the negative stigmas flourished vividly in my mind. Here I was, a business man on Wall Street in Manhattan, hiding out between subway cars to take an urgent dump. It was insane and it made me crazy, I used to s--t my pants two to three times a week and even wore diapers.

My career as a broker had ended a year after 9/11. On that fateful day, I watched the horrific scene unfold from my TV. Annually, I took that week off to commemorate the loss of my father who died on September 11, 1986. Watching the news in horror of the survivors walking for miles on the expressway, all I could think about was how devastated I would have been as I tried to get home without crapping on myself. I continued with medicinal treatments until I finally hit the brick wall in April 2006—twenty-four long years since my original IBS diagnosis.

The J-pouch surgery was my miracle waiting to happen, but soon pure acid was coming out of my bottom and my butt was burnt to a crisp; I couldn't touch it without extreme pain. I formerly used the bathroom fifteen to twenty times daily; with the J-pouch, it increased to twenty to thirty times a day. It was no life and with my back against the wall, I called my surgeon, "I can't live like this anymore, we have to do something." He admitted me to perform a permanent ileostomy.

Dying emotionally and physically, I pushed my wife and my children away. Wanting them to let me go, my only comfort was in knowing I had secured them with enough insurance. Life was slipping through my fingers into a downward spiral and then came the introduction of life-saving Zoloft in my life.

Within five months of surgery, I moved from my family and rented a room in a hostel. We were transients, a houseful of thirty to forty people that had fallen off life's tracks. With a shared bathroom and shower, I had a studio with a sink, microwave, and bed—sparse, but all I needed as I adapted to my ostomy. For the first time in years, I had full control and found I could use my private sink to clean and empty my pouch. Without accidents, I begin to appreciate my ostomy.

Within weeks I got a blockage and headed to the hospital brought by a wonderful, wacky girl from the hostel. Over time we shared our stories, and I wanted to be with her; I was yearning for intimacy. Even though I was scared about how things would work, being in this place where no one knew me made me feel a bit more comfortable. She was attractive, lived next to me, and we shared a bathroom. One night while watching TV together, I said, "Let me share with you what I look like and what I've been through." She agreed, and I was fairly comfortable pulling my pants down to show her my ostomy; I wasn't naked, but I felt vulnerable. Conversation flowed and I felt something might happen, not knowing or caring what came about, my heart started to pound. I didn't disrobe entirely.

"Leave your pants off. It's not so bad—you look great," she said adding several much needed compliments. She was the first woman I laid with semi-naked since my ostomy. While we were touching each other, I found with the antidepressants, my ability to have an erection was gone. I gave her pleasure; she hadn't had sex in a long time, and allowed herself to freely let go and have orgasms like crazy. She wanted to give me pleasure in return but I wouldn't let her near me for lack of an erection. Her excitement added to mine and to my surprise I ejaculated while being completely flaccid. It reminded me of my first sexual encounter as a young man. I was totally baffled how at age forty-eight, I had an orgasm without anyone touching me. She fell asleep in five minutes while I laid there and thought, *Oh my God this is amazing; what just happened?*

It was too soon to know if the non-erection was a result of the ostomy, the medicine, or my mental state. I visited the doctor to check my testosterone levels and after finding the Zoloft affected my libido, I was allowed to wean from it to see how things progressed.

The next intimate setting was with a dear friend whose husband had left her. We were close and she loved my words and my truthful conversations about life. We could talk about anything and we did.

"You are so attractive," I said to her, leaning closer.

"You are too," she replied.

In this surreal moment, I leaned over and kissed her.

"Did you just kiss me? Are you sure you want to do that?" she asked.

I thought to myself, *Yes!*

It soon got more passionate even though I lacked my sexual confidence, and I wasn't 100 percent yet. Three months had passed since that first encounter, and I was delightfully pleased when I found I was able to have an orgasm with an erection, albeit not for long.

Living in New York, divorce is difficult without disrupting our children's lives, and my wife and I have not filed yet. I feel badly that my daughter lived through my steroid use with ulcerative colitis and saw an angry dad for many years. With no chance of getting back to the life I had with my wife, we honor the fact that we made two beautiful children. We credit the illness with the demise of the last twelve years of our marriage. I once told her she was crazy for staying with me through all the misery and surgeries and thanked her for giving me her best shot. In the end, it was just too much; it had robbed us of what we once were. We have a healthy separation and are amicable. I like her boyfriend and he likes me as a friend and it is all okay. We put in twenty-two years together and now we wish for the other to be happy. It just won't be as before, with us being man and wife.

Venturing to Match.com a year after the ileostomy, I met someone and appreciated her beauty, intellect, and her acceptance of me. She had suffered in her marriage too, and we happily frolicked like teenagers for a year. My pouch was never an issue in our sexual experimentation, and it had dawned on me that I am a strong male, here to stay, and women out there will love me. Women seem to have amazing coping skills, and from what I read and hear, more so than the male when it comes to a partner in this journey.

As a result of that year-long relationship, my confidence was secure when a coworker and I became interested in each other. We hooked up. While making passionate love under the stars, my pouch fell off. Within thirty seconds after feeling for my pouch and reattaching it, we got back to business as if nothing had happened and it was good.

Another wardrobe malfunction occurred when I was involved with a nurse who understood my medical journey. However, early on, when hands started moving and progressing down below, her hand went under my ostomy belt and pulled the pouch off in its entirety. It was a show stopper as I ran around her house naked, went to the basement with its cold floors, did a load of laundry, and went back upstairs to shower, hopped back into bed, and we got on with it. If anyone would have said these things would happen and it *wouldn't* affect me *and* I'd be able to laugh at myself, I would have thought they were crazy.

I want to make the rest of my body attractive. It may be psychological, a need to compensate for the ostomy—so be it. I work out doing yoga, spin classes, work with weights, and try to be physically fit. I want the woman to be attracted to me and say, "What pouch?"

I love to blog on MeetAnOstoMate.com. and feel sad when a woman writes, "*What can I do to make him want me?*" The truth is it is never the ostomy that's the issue, even though it gets the brunt of the blame. If the relationship is not working, the ostomy becomes the scapegoat. Most likely things were already deteriorating and the ostomy becomes the excuse that pushes the relationship over the cliff.

I've had many dates where I've been rejected. If the first date went great and I was attracted, I would let her know early. I felt obligated to share my journey. Telling women I was ill for a long time wasn't enough. So I would have them guess what illness. They would often respond with, "Alcoholism?" "Cancer?" I soon learned guessing would take them into crazy places. It would ruin the moment, so I stopped. The best time to tell them was different for each person. A nurse or someone from the medical establishment might be told sooner than a person who has no medical knowledge. I thought I read people fairly well, the kissing, the hand holding, and their eyes would be kind, but there would be no follow-up date. I guess I had more to learn.

The first two women that rejected me saddened me. There were other women who, when they touched my pants and heard them crinkle, there would be no more phone calls. Sometimes I was surprised if we kissed well and seemed compatible, and then no more interest. I would ask, "What happened?" One woman simply said she decided to go in another direction.

It has taught me that it's all okay and their reactions are normal, too. Understanding of ostomy is still foreign to most people; they can't begin to comprehend the freedom the pouch has brought to me. I still can't believe it, and I want to do my part to change the stigmas—until then the reactions, both good and bad, will continue.

I can tell you in a thousand ways how the ostomy has given me a new life. One favorite being the lifelong friends made through the UOAA as well as my local chapter. Coming full circle, I look at my illness as a gift. Previously, I lived my life trying to be perfect and that path was killing me. I believe my quest for impossible perfection manifested itself in my illness—I never felt worthy. When I became an ostomate and technically became imperfect, it allowed me to relax and to learn to live with my imperfections, which was a transformational event for me.

Being a fifty-two-year-old ostomate, I still desire to have a long-term relationship and a strong connection to a woman, preferably someone who has embraced her own amazing journey living with an ostomy. I think it would be magical to share this gift of life.

———— ⑧ ————

LONG DISTANCE DATING
Nancy Olesky

Before I was five years old, I had seven abdominal surgeries. Born six weeks prematurely, I've had an ileal conduit (urinary diversion) since before I was two years old. I had many internal complications and one turned out to be a bad bladder. I have been wearing an ostomy bag most of my fifty years of life and have led a pretty normal life while going to school, despite being quiet and shy.

I wasn't into dating in school, but when I started working, I dated a couple of people. When I would finally tell them about the ostomy, they would back off. Consequently, I didn't date much at all. Thank God for the Internet because I came across the website MeetAnOstoMate.com and signed up. There I met a man from the UK, and I started writing to him. We had a lot in common with the same kind of ostomies since childhood and are both the youngest in our families.

We have been writing for about six years now, and he has visited me twice. We have had a great friendship and a sexual relationship as well. We feel very comfortable with each other as we exchange ideas on ostomy supplies and have a good time together. We write to each other every day and have been a source of support as well, not only about the ostomy similarities but everyday things such as job loss and other issues. I currently suffer from short bowel syndrome due to all the abdominal surgeries, but I try to carry on. I live in the bathroom some days, but as the doctors say, "Learn to live with it."

He has brought me out of my shell about my body and changed the way I look at myself and made me feel a bit more normal.

———— ⊛ ————

MY BAG ISN'T ME
MATT (ANONYMOUS)

A few weeks before I started my sophomore year in college, I got an ileostomy due to ulcerative colitis. College was a rough time to get a bag. I was away from home and away from the support of my family and most of my friends. I went to a huge university, but I was painfully shy and had made only one new friend in the two semesters I had been there. This was a few years before the Internet came around, so I knew of no one else my age who could relate to having this nasty, smelly bag.

I thought everybody could tell what was under my shirt, and I believed deep down they thought I was gross because of it. I was embarrassed to have it. The accidents could be humiliating. Plus, I felt the weight of shame as having the bag broke two social taboos.

The first taboo applied against having feces anywhere in public but in a toilet, and certainly not attached to you as you walk around. The second taboo applied specifically to a young man, the taboo against being physically imperfect.

There is still a lot of caveman lurking in the genetics of college-aged kids, and a young woman's genes pushes her towards the guy who appears strong enough to hunt the lion and defend the cave from the wildebeest, or whatever they defended caves from back then. A coed is more apt to see the starting quarterback as if he's Conan the Barbarian more than the skinny sophomore with the glasses and the pooh bag.

Needless to say, dating was a terrifying thought. I felt alone, and it didn't help that my guy friends were trading off their hook-up stories while I sat there knowing I couldn't so much as get a girl's attention. It also didn't help that occasionally I would hear a friend say how glad they were not to have to be me.

I did try to ask out girls from time to time, but that, too, was a disaster. It took me six calendar years to get through college from both the obligatory major change, as well as the obligatory missing-an-entire-year-due-to-illness that everyone with IBD (Inflammatory Bowel Disease) or an ostomy seems to have. In those six years, I went out with one girl, and she could have gotten a part-time job as modeling sin—not cute. The last laugh was on me, though, as she dumped me after a week and went back with her ex without telling me. I must have asked out a dozen girls in college, and with the exception of that one girl, was turned down by each one. I kept telling myself it must have been my bag.

But in my last year of college I had a revelation: Every girl I asked out on a date had known I had a bag before I asked them out, most of them because *I had told them*. I never stopped to think about how I was so focused on how terrible I thought having a bag was that my attitude about my bag was permeating its way into my personality. And, in retrospect, I never paid attention to the girls who were flirting with me, because I had assumed they would never be interested in me. Girls never had the chance to see me first, because I was making them see the bag first. Girls weren't avoiding me because I had a bag of pooh; they were avoiding me because *I was depressing to be around!* Who the heck wants to date a depressing bag of pooh?

That was the point things started to slowly change for me. I began ignoring my bag and started focusing on my life instead, and as an unintended consequence, women started hitting on me. I was attractive, smart, confident (by this time), and funny, and they were taking notice. By the time I was in my mid-twenties, it began to be a bit of a problem because most of them weren't my type, and I was never comfortable turning girls down. I hit upon what I thought was an awesome solution. I figured that if before girls didn't want me because of my bag, I'll just sneak it into conversation, and *voila!*— instant female disinterest, and I didn't have to be the bad guy. I high-fived myself.

What I found out instead was the opposite. Because they got to know me first as a person, my having a bag made them *more interested* in me because suddenly I was set apart from other guys as being courageous and having depth and sensitivity. I also met several young ladies who were quick to voice their intentions with me, always leaving me at a loss for words.

Eventually I was asked out by a girl I thought I could have a dating relationship with (remember, I was still very shy), and it quickly got intimate. I think my bag was trying to tell me something about her by the way it leaked on her naked body three times. My bag had never let me down in love.

I finally met the woman I would marry, and again, I said nothing about my bag at first. I let her get to know me as a person, and she tells me that on her own she figured out I had it. As hard as it was to do at first, ignoring my bag in favor of paying attention to my life was the best thing I ever did. My bag wasn't me; it just took me a while to figure that out.

———— ✆ ————

MR. BLUE EYES
MORGAN (ANONYMOUS)

I was younger, wilder, and reeling from the pain of a failed marriage. I had gone to a party at a guy's apartment. I recall that I was the only girl there—how lame was that party. Someone knocked on the door and the host asked me to get the door, so I did. Standing in the doorway were four young sailors. One of them had those eyes, the ones you can just fall into and not get out of. I was lost—hook, line, and sinker—gone. That poor guy that invited me over, my date, never stood another chance. How I remembered my voice to invite them in I'm not sure, but suddenly after introductions, I hear the host say, "Morgan, this is Nick," then "Oh, you two probably already know each other, he's Roger's old roommate."

I said, "You're that Nick."

To which he said, "You're that Morgan."

We spent the rest of the night talking like old friends; I caught him up on what my friend Roger had been up to since Nick had been out to sea, all the while trying to figure out a way to see him again. I was on a tight schedule. I had another date later. Three dates in one night, and I met Mr. Blue Eyes—it was a banner night.

The next day Roger brought Nick to my work and invited me over later. More talking, and after we left Roger's, we talked until the wee hours of the morning. Somehow plans were made that in three days, we were getting a motel room. Meanwhile, Roger could not figure out why we were so tired. But every night after we left him, we talked and talked, but I never told him about my surgery. I wanted him so badly I didn't want to scare him—like waiting would help.

The hotel night came; it was winter and snowing. He got out to get the room at the first place, and came back to the car to report, "No vacancy." At the next place I went in to check—success! I went back to the car with a key for room number sixty-nine. We got a laugh out of that. I would not advise anyone to wait until you get to this point before telling someone you have an ostomy. My only excuse is that he was so darn cute, or the eyes got to me, I really don't know. But anyhow it was do or die time and I had to say, "Wait— stop, I have to tell you something first." He looked at me with those gorgeous eyes and said, "I know, Roger already told me." All I could think was *Thank you, Roger.*

---- ⊛ ----

KEEP LOOKING
Marcella Taylor-Billing

Things changed for my husband before I had surgery; we shared the same bed but were no longer intimate. I was too sick to worry about it, although it was nice to cuddle up. I had my ostomy in February 1986 and was happily married when I had surgery. When I came home from the hospital, my husband had made up the spare room for me, telling me I would be more comfortable in there. I, too, thought that it would be for the best, at least for a few weeks, giving us both time to adjust. Five years down the line I was still in the spare room. I did try to go back to our bedroom, but it was not what he wanted and he was shocked that I desired that. All I wanted was a normal life. Our arguments became more and more frequent till in the end I left him, and we divorced in '92.

I met another man, a bit of a whirlwind, and before I knew it, we were married. It didn't last long, not even a year. I think I went along with it just to prove to my first husband that there was life after an ostomy.

I was on my own again so I moved to London. I needed to work. I am a chef, and I lived in one of the big five-star hotels, always going with someone out on the town and having loads of fun but never meeting anyone in particular.

I longed for a partner. I was fifty and sold my house in Northampton and bought a narrow boat to live on, thinking that would attract a nice guy. I imagined we would cruise the canals stopping where and when we wanted—it was a dream. Instead, I met a young man of thirty-five and we had two lovely years together filled with laughter. His ex kept telling him I was too old. She didn't want him but was not happy for us to be together either. At least I still have the boat. I had gone looking for a piece of property, but they were all too expensive. Looking through a local paper one day, I found a boat for sale. I wanted my own front door after living in a small room for too long, so thought I would give it a go.

She was a bit of a wreck, so I bought some power tools and, with the help of my sons, we started work. She is now a cozy home; she still has no engine but is really warm in the winter. It's so lovely when spring comes around to see the swans with their cygnets and all the baby ducks, too—the wild life is amazing, the kingfisher are beautiful. I love my boat and hope I can live on it forever.

My stoma has never stopped me from doing anything, I have been to Australia twice, many places in the USA, and now I would just like to share time with a nice, special man.

After my last relationship, I got involved with a guy who ripped me off to the tune of £4,000, so I find it difficult to trust. I pray to God that someday I will be with someone who will respect and care for me as much as I will care for him. Then I will no longer be on my own, as life sometimes gets lonely when you are retired, and it's fun to share this beauty of nature.

———— ✆ ————

GO AHEAD AND GET PHYSICAL
Kelly Livingston

When I decided I was ready to put myself back out there, about a year after my surgery for ileostomy due to FAP (Familial Adenomatous Polyposis), I decided online dating was the best avenue for me. It didn't come without its share of heartache and lessons learned with new tactics of ways to navigate the dating pool. I hoped it would help me cut through a lot of the crap, literally and figuratively.

My intro line for my profile is, "First let me say that I come with baggage; I would be lying if I didn't. Who doesn't have some at this point in one's life? But, rest assured, it's packed." It definitely drew interest, but many never truly figured out what I actually meant.

I met a lot of interesting men, some nice, others still licking wounds, some with addictive habits that, after dating a while, basically told me I should feel lucky to be with them, as there aren't many guys out there that would want to put up with a woman with a bag. They were just that—guys. I would later find out, it takes a gentleman to see the wonderful woman I am and not my bag. There were a few players that were only looking for one thing, and I have since learned you look for that on Craigslist.

I learned to see my ileostomy as my ace in the hole to see what the men were really interested in. Despite using my ostomy as my guard, it was obvious some men really just wanted sex, plain and simple. The very first guy I dated said all the right things, but once he got what he wanted, *and* found out about my ostomy, disappeared. Initially I was devastated, wallowed in self-pity for a couple months, and then decided I needed to put myself back out there, hoping for a better representation of what I thought, and believed, most men were.

On a third date with one guy, I needed to have the "bag talk," and he honestly had no idea what an ostomy was. I drove home trying to wrap my head around the fact that I couldn't determine if this guy thought I was an alien, a leper, or a transsexual. He actually asked me if what I was trying to tell him is that I still have a penis.

From that experience, I decided I needed to "out" my baggage early, before either side became too invested emotionally. Full disclosure is the best policy. We, my bag and I, are a package deal, and I am accepting of the fact there are plenty of men that can't deal with it. Let's just part ways amicably and move on. A few of them have become great friends and rather protective of me in a big brother way.

In the past four years, I have met and dated more than twenty-five men. Some never progressed beyond the initial meet, or as one guy coined it, after a week of many lengthy e-mail exchanges, the coffee interview. My friends, both married and shy, and insecure single ones, were living vicariously through me, who looked as if I had plans with a different guy every night. Who has the energy for that?

It's a good idea to do something physically active on the first date. Once I've shared my ostomy story, some guys in the past presumed it disabled me. Having an ostomy doesn't disable me—it truly enables me to be an active participant in my life again. With my current boyfriend, we went hiking, stopped, sat on a rock, and had takeout lunch. We started talking about life and what it throws at you and how we choose to handle it. He admitted he didn't know much about ostomies, but he also didn't make an excuse to end the date rapidly.

He contacted me the next morning, apologizing for the short notice, and asked if I was available to go scrambling (climbing rocks without the aid of ropes or other extreme gear). I had never done that before and that date lasted more than six hours. As he dropped me off at my home, he admitted he had spent the night before searching the Internet and reading about ostomies. He said he didn't realize there were different types and some were temporary. That he was interested enough to research on his own spoke volumes of him as a gentleman.

He wasn't afraid of my ostomy; he was more concerned that intimacy would hurt. After weeks of dating and assuring him there were no worries, we took our relationship to the next level. Our first leak together occurred on our first roughing it camping trip. No running water, no port-a-potty, nothing!

We decided to explore one of many canyons we came across and reached the end of the canyon when he decided to get frisky. One thing led to another and I found my bag caught between a rock and a hard place and the rock won. We hiked out before the bag pulled completely away.

He likes to snuggle after making love while we sleep. I am always hesitant, fearing an appliance malfunction, but gave in the other night, under the false security of having just changed my bag and wafer. I had secured the new one in place and had on a special intimacy wrap covering my bag. When I awoke feeling moisture on my hand, I tossed back the covers to find poop oozing out from between the wrap and my abdomen, semi-dried on his back. It was all over the bedding, soaking through to the mattress pad. I leapt out of bed, and initially wet a washcloth with warm water, and tried to gently wipe off his back, hoping to not have to wake him, until I realized the full scope of the damage to be addressed at 1:00 in the morning. I gently woke him, think-ing this is the end of a wonderful, normal relationship. He woke up, helped strip the bed, remade it, and carried the bedding to the laundry room. Any lingering doubts about what that incident did to our relationship vanished the next morning with a simple phone text, "Snuggling with you last night was wonderful."

———— ✿ ————

LOVE ME, LOVE PRISCI
ROSANA E. PAZ

I was born in Maracaibo, Venezuela, and moved to Caracas to follow my dream—to be famous, rich, and travel around the world. In 2002, my large intestine was in trouble and the sigmoid was removed, which was a huge mistake. I had the second surgery, a colostomy, and J-pouch because my large intestine was paralyzed. It is a congenital syndrome. It did not work due to the small intestine having the same syndrome, so later in the year the ileostomy came into my life.

Before the ileostomy, my doctor, who was already my friend, asked me if I would agree with surgery. I remember asking him, "How much time do I have without surgery?"

He replied, "Without surgery, maybe three to four months to live, and with surgery, at least two years."

I remember thinking *I can make love many more times in two years than in three to four months, so let's go do the surgery if my dad can pay for it.* I did not have insurance and was in the USA on a tourist visa.

Since I can remember, I have always been the kind of woman that draws attention. Wherever I walk, everybody turns their faces to look, either because of how I dress or how I talk. It has helped me to have people around me, especially men. To be honest, I took advantage of that. At the same time, it made me a little emotionally dependent to always need to have a partner in life.

When the ileostomy came, called "Prisci," I was sharing time with someone for years, but soon realized he wanted to be my nurse more than my partner. I didn't feel good about it; it wasn't right for me and my needs as a woman.

He moved back to Venezuela, and in April 2003, my search started for something different. At a friend's suggestion, I went to Match.com, where I met a lot of people. I also learned a lot about how to handle Prisci and how to make people love Prisci before me—that became my first priority.

At that point, I had other things I had to deal with—my hysterectomy, no babies, and scars with my mastectomy, breast implants, and breast cancer scars, and even though I was looking good, it was a huge worry for me.

I was honest on my profile and wrote, "I am very smart, fine, well-educated, professional, funny, and attractive with a special beauty. I am looking for a special man capable of sharing difficult times and one who believes in second chances in life with no babies in the future."

That gave me the opportunity to talk easily about special beauty and second chances in life. At first people got surprised about my looks. I am a Latin woman, with green eyes, long black hair with a tan, skinny, but with muscles and that helped me a little bit to distract them about the real stuff that was inside—the bag, the scars, the implants.

On my first date I was not brave enough to talk about it. He was nice, but I did not feel that it would go further than just going out. After a few dates, he got more interested in me than I was in him. I really used Prisci to make him run away without hurting his feelings. I told him I have a very important thing to share that will change his feelings about me. He asked me, "What is that? Did you lie to me? Do you have kids?"

I said, "No, I don't have kids, but it is worse than that because kids you could have them go away to have fun or go to a vacation by ourselves. This has to be with me forever."

He was in shock when I removed my clothes a little bit and showed Prisci to him. His eyes were out of his face, and he said, "I can't deal with that."

I replied, "Sorry, then, because I can't take off Prisci while I am with you. She has to be with me always to be able to be alive." It was over.

On my second date I decided to talk about Prisci right away. I was pleased he did not care about Prisci at all. We had plenty of free time to see if we wanted to be together in a formal way, but it did not work out. I just wanted to prove to myself that everything could be normal even with Prisci, but I wasn't ready for the commitment.

It was in June 2003, when I read about a handsome man, but too picky, in Match.com. I decided to take the first step and sent an e-mail to him. His profile said, "If you have children or want them and if you are not petite and weigh more than 105 pounds, don't bother answering."

When I saw that, I said to myself: *I weigh ninety-nine pounds, don't have babies, and can't have babies, so that is me.*

We started chatting and talking by phone, and the next month we met. He did not know anything about my stuff, so I decided to tell him everything that day. He was much more handsome in person than the picture, and it made me a little afraid to talk. We went to a fine Japanese (my favorite food) restaurant in Orlando, and I had a lot of sake first and then I talked.

I told him what I said on my profile about special beauty needed further explanation before going further. It was time for me to tell him I had implants, I had a hysterectomy done, and I have a bag called "Prisci" that is an ileostomy attached to my beautiful belly, to be able to be alive and have a normal life as long as God wants.

"I know how picky you are about physical stuff, but this is me and this is what I have. If you don't like it or you cannot handle it—okay we can be friends and that's it."

He told me to please stop and let him talk. "I have to love all of that because I want to love you and I don't want to lose you ... period! Nothing else to talk about ..."

My next proof to see if he was the right one for me and Prisci was when I had him watch while I changed my bag. "I want to know if something happens and I am not able to change Prisci myself, you can do it."

I knew then he wasn't concerned about having Prisci between us. We moved in together and got married, but eventually we went our separate ways. Now, here again I am starting over, and I'll keep going. I keep working on my career, keep painting, and looking for a relationship to share life with somebody again.

———— ✿ ————

OVERCOMING FEAR OF REJECTION
MICHAEL R. (ANONYMOUS)

The summer after graduating from high school I found out I had ulcerative colitis and was presented with ostomy surgery or death. I ended up having an ileostomy—they took everything out and closed the anus. I hadn't been sexually active in high school and was still a virgin at that time. They may have suggested counseling, but I just wanted to go home.

I was able to start college the following quarter with hardly anyone but immediate family knowing about the surgery and only one friend from high school. I had nurses tell them I didn't want visitors and they put a sign up to that effect. I figured my new friends at college didn't need to know either.

I didn't know what to do with the first girl I got close to. We dated nine months, and I knew she wondered if there was something wrong with her. I wanted to be physical with her; I trusted her—I just didn't know how to go about it. Mom's advice was if she didn't accept it, she's probably not the person for me.

I wimped out. I sent her a letter. I didn't want to face her. The letter explained the surgery to her and that she meant a lot to me and if she didn't feel comfortable being with me I would understand. I told her I wanted to be closer to her because we had expressed love for one another and also I knew she wanted to be closer physically. I didn't want to push her off, but the fear of facing it was too strong.

She called when she received the letter and said it wasn't that big of a deal. She wanted to know more about it. I didn't even know how to explain it; a lot of it was still a mystery to me. I showed her and she didn't react. That baffled my mind. I still hadn't really accepted it so when she didn't react negatively, it shocked me. To her it was no big deal; to me it was a huge deal.

To this day, thirty years later, I still think it's disheartening. It baffles me to use humor; I have gotten a lot better since I was eighteen. I know it saved my life, but I'm still not very good with it.

That first woman was very accepting; we had sex that night. I remember before the surgery that the doctor said I could become impotent; it didn't even cross my mind—everything happened in a blur. If that had occurred, it would have been a whole other ball game. Luckily, all went well and we dated for about two years before we broke up and moved on.

I have been sexually involved with eight different women, and they have been very accepting. I have had one-night stands that turned into longer relationships.

Eventually, I went to see a therapist. I was asked, "Ever had anyone reject you because of your ostomy? You are just waiting for it to happen."

It turned out that I was waiting for someone to validate my wrong thinking so I could say, "See, I told you."

He's asked me different questions about my fears. My fears were campgrounds and one big shower room.

The thing I have learned from the relationships is that the ostomy is such a small part of me—after I told them, some of them even forgot. The intimacy has gone well.

I fight having an ostomy; I still try to figure out ways to hide it. I used to get a pouch cover and I felt it added more attention. I looked at the smaller bags and didn't like those either.

I was asked, "Have you ever gone skinny dipping?"

I said no.

"Let's go find a lake that's really quiet."

It was freeing and for a lack of a better word, I felt normal. I felt happy and it was exciting.

Because of having an ostomy, I get to know people on a different level; it's created the person I am—a lot more compassionate.

I got a piece of advice from the first girl to not wait as long as I did with her. With the last woman I got close to, I handled it differently. We drove to a spot overlooking the river up high, which looks over the city. "I need to tell you something." I made things huge and built it up so much. "Have you ever heard of ulcerative colitis? I had it when I was younger. I have a pouch on the side," and left it at that.

In amazement, she said, "Okay, maybe I should tell you something about myself."

We told each other our true confessions. We didn't sleep together right away; we waited a few weeks before we had sex. At times I'm disappointed around sex, especially when I can't be as spontaneous if I have to change the bag. I like to make sure it's dark with candles in the corner versus bright like on the beach.

The biggest difference in my life for the ostomy is Devrom tablets. The odor was a huge thing. I take the tablets around meals. It's like a new world opened up for me. I can stay at people's houses without worrying about the odor anymore. Lots of opportunities are coming my way and since I have been more honest, there seems to be a lot of good changes.

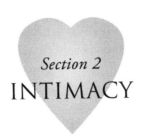

Section 2
INTIMACY

My friends tell me I have an intimacy problem. But they don't really know me.
—Garry Shandling

Passion is the quickest to develop, and the quickest to fade. Intimacy develops more slowly and commitment more gradually still.
—Robert Sternberg

While growing up I had a very romantic idea of intimacy. I thought my husband would come home with roses; we would have a candlelight dinner, give each other languorous body massages, and then feed each other strawberries dipped in chocolate. I am sure that happens for some people and lucky them. The reality is I do get a rose when he changes the oil on the car (they give them away at the car dealer), we haven't had a candlelit dinner since we ate at a restaurant in the Bahamas where I don't think they wanted us to see the delicacy we were eating—sheep tongue, and body massages are few and far between because we are too exhausted. The other weird thing is that I never even liked strawberries.

I did have a good role model of my father teasing my mother affectionately and of them making breakfasts together and him popping the bubbles on her pancakes and she would act all mad about it. He would tease her out of her exhaustion and frustration at her children, grab her and pull her onto his lap, and hold her long enough to make her laugh. Intimacy to me was moments like that—a total acceptance of the other person.

I remember one Sunday a few years ago, my husband and I were peacefully enjoying reading the paper and relaxing on a Sunday morning. Looking at the two of us soaking in the sun through the porch windows, no one would have guessed we were just recovering from a colossal fight where hurtful words were exchanged earlier in the week that could never be taken back.

We were still licking our wounds as I decided to put in a new Celine Dion CD that Bahgat had just purchased. We enjoyed it and continued reading until we noticed the new CD got stuck on a song. Ironically, it was a duet with Luciano Pavarotti and Celine called, "I Hate You, Then I Love You." As we replayed it to get it unstuck, we had to laugh as we listened more closely to the lyrics. It was about how our partner drives us crazy and we'd rather be alone. It went on to say how impossible it is to live with the other but how impossible it would be to live without them. It's a great song about the angst between the couple and ends up with words that many of us can relate to—I hate you, and I love you and never want anyone else but you. It's a fine line sometimes between those strong feelings and it summed up our emotions of the week.

It was doubly funny when we were called a short time later and asked if we would give a talk at my church on marriage around Valentine's Day. I told the person that asked us that I didn't think we were the appropriate couple for the job and explained how our marriage had hit a tough time recently. Instead, she said, "Perfect—that is what I want you to tell people. Who can't relate to that?" We thought about it and even had some fun doing it. Bahgat pretended he was Luciano, and I took the part of Celine and we lip-synched this song right into the hearts of the couples present, just as Celine and Luciano did for us.

Intimacy has so many meanings and in the stories that follow, you'll get a sense of what it means for each contributor and their partners through the challenging times dealing with an ostomy.

———— ✆ ————

YOU ARE BEAUTIFUL
Veralynne Malone

While my first husband accepted the ileostomy I had in 1980 and the ups and downs one can have with them, our marriage ended five years later. I figured no one else would be attracted to me and that I would become an old lady, loved by no one, bitter and reclusive.

That same year I had a new neighbor move in next door to me. He was single and really good looking. Not thinking of love or anything, I tried to be neighborly by offering coffee and such while he was getting his mobile home set up. He was the quiet kind, and I wasn't sure how he felt about me being his neighbor. After he got settled in, he went back to Texas to get his personal belongings and his dog that he left there while he had been deployed on a seven-month Mediterranean naval cruise. When he came back, he warned me that his dog didn't take kindly to strangers, and he wasn't sure how she would react to my son and me.

As time went on, we chatted and became friends and I befriended his dog Pepper. I fed her treats and leftovers when he was on duty and made sure she had water. To this day he says that Pepper fell in love with me first. When my first marriage fell apart, I never thought I'd find love again, but before it went too far, I had to explain my ileostomy to him.

The first thing he asked was, "Are you happy with yourself?

I said, "Sure, I am alive and that's all that really matters.

He said, "If you can love yourself, I can love you, too."

My son and I moved in with him while my divorce was becoming final. The first time we made love I was scared to death. I made sure my bag was empty, that I was clean and smelled good. I had also made some cute little bag covers and had on my red one that night. He made me leave the light on, and I really hated it, but afterward I was glad he did because he was able to see me as I really was. He kept saying, "You are beautiful" and that was all that mattered to me.

We will soon be celebrating our twenty-fourth wedding anniversary, and while everything hasn't been roses, my ileostomy has never been an issue. So for those women out there who think they aren't beautiful, know that you are, and you just need the right man to see it.

---— ☙ ——---

PATIENCE BRINGS CLOSENESS
Andy Fletcher

Before I had a panproctocolectomy and ileostomy in 2008, I enjoyed a very active sex life with my wife, Julie. We were warned by the surgeon that the operation carried a risk of damaging erectile tissue. I felt I had no alternative but to proceed with the operation. I had suffered for years with pain, embarrassing accidents, and ill health.

It was no great surprise in recovering from the operation that I discovered the damage was done. For a few months after the operation, I was in no mood to attempt sex, as recovery was slow and painful, but when we were ready and tried to have sex, we discovered I was suffering from erectile dysfunction and the mood was lost.

A doctor prescribed Viagra, followed by Cialis, and although these worked to a certain extent, we found the entire process very clinical. There was no passion involved, which is the whole point in the first place. A year later, I found I can gain an erection without the need for drugs. However, it is not sustained, and I lose it quicker than I gain it. I fear this is now the end of our sex life as it is—although if I am being honest, we have not tried since. Fear of failure is very strong, and it is difficult to remove the stigma from my mind.

Throughout this ordeal, my wife has been totally understanding and very patient. She feels my frustration. She is not pushing for resolution on this. We both know we will try again one day, but Julie is taking a side step and will not pressure me until I feel I am ready.

I do not regret the operation one little bit. It gave me back a quality of life that I had forgotten about. I am only forty-seven years old, and the potential loss of a sex life is hard to accept, but in a round-about way, it has brought my wife and me closer together. We spend more time together doing things we would not have normally done. For example, I enjoy the peace of sea fishing. Julie always comes with me to either try fishing herself, or just to read a book on a quiet beach. In return, we tend to go out for meals more. We talk more, and watch TV less. We socialize with friends more, but the largest change I have noticed in our relationship is that we enjoy each other's company more. There is a level of trust that, although always there, has been extended. I know my wife loves me, and she knows I love her. That makes up for a lack of a sex life for the time being.

We both know the time will come again when we will attempt to make love. I am unsure about trying for fear of failure, and Julie has remained patient. This wonderful patience of hers has brought us much closer together and that's good.

——— ⊛ ———

100 PERCENT LOVE
ANITA AND WILLIAM SUMMERS

ANITA

From the time I was a young child, I was often ill. I was only ten years old when I was first diagnosed with ulcerative colitis, sick again briefly at age eighteen, and then was symptom-free until I was thirty-six. I became increasingly ill for the next eleven years, and then lost thirty pounds in four weeks. I was literally dying of malnutrition and dehydration because my colon was too shredded to absorb much of anything anymore.

Hospitalized to stop the bleeding, I was treated for the bleeding until the diagnosis came that my colon and rectum were too far gone, which resulted in the need for a permanent ileostomy.

The first time the WOC Nurse came in to teach me about the bag change before discharge, I wanted my husband to leave the room, fearing the emotional risk of me seeing him get grossed out. He insisted on staying. I felt disgusting and assumed everyone else would think I was too, but he just stood there, totally calm while she removed my bag and exposed my new surgical site and stoma.

Afterward I was crying, "How come you didn't run screaming from the room?"

"I have gutted a lot of deer," he said impassively, and he was just grateful I was alive.

After we got home, he helped me cut and place the bag the first couple of times, then he disengaged, never to be involved in any way again.

Before my surgery I had been in so much pain for years that intercourse had been difficult to impossible, but he refused to do anything else to be physically intimate. He would frequently get very angry and blame me for ruining his sex life, claiming that was the cause of the fact that he was crabby most of the time.

My symptoms got worse when I was under severe stress, so things went from bad to worse. Once I had the surgery and could enjoy intercourse again, he was happier, sex was frequent and comfortable, and the bag was never an issue. We had many other serious problems, though, and when I was well enough to manage on my own, we separated after fewer than five years of marriage.

Four weeks later William and I met at church. I was instantly attracted to him, and we sat together during the service. Afterward we talked for about an hour and a half, and in that first conversation, I was totally frank with William about some personal issues.

"I was really sick; my colon was shredded and had to be taken out, and I have an ostomy. Do you know what that is?"

"No."

"Well, I have a bag attached to my abdomen and that's where I s--t now," I said nervously.

WILLIAM

When Anita told me she had a bag, in my mind I thought it was a big bag about ten to fourteen inches and one that could hold ten pounds of s--t. You don't have any idea until you see one. That didn't matter anyway; I knew I was going to marry Anita the moment I saw her, which was a little confusing because I was engaged to someone else at the time. We met in February, but I waited until summer (and after I broke up with my fiancée) to tell her I wanted to marry her. A lot had to happen for both of us before that could transpire.

ANITA

Before meeting William, I had been playing an online game for a few years and had come to care very deeply for someone from Scotland whom I had met on the game. We talked on webcam together, and at one point after my separation, he wanted to see my stoma. I was very scared, but I went to the bathroom, removed the bag, cleaned up, and set the camera at desk level.

He started laughing, "I have no idea what you were worried about, Anita, this is nothing."

I was so relieved he wasn't freaked out about it; it was a hugely liberating moment for me. Until then the only men who had seen my stoma were my surgeon and my estranged husband, and at that moment I understood it was possible for other men to be okay with it as well.

One of the reasons I didn't get divorced sooner was because I struggled wondering who would want me with my physical appearance. This concern had been drummed into my head countless times by my husband when he was being emotionally abusive, "No one else is going to want you with that bag and those scars."

After we separated, someone from my hometown was on my mind. We had become very good friends over the previous ten years and had grown to love one another. After I had separated and met William, this hometown man and I had been talking a lot. I was sure nothing could ever come of it, but I felt I had to resolve anything I had wondered about from that relationship before I could move on with a fully open heart, so I went back to my hometown and saw him.

He hadn't had sex in five years, was a doctor, and didn't care at all about my ostomy. He was just insanely happy and grateful to be together after all those years of us being very interested in each other, but not being able to express it or act on it out of respect for our marriages. After spending the weekend with him, I knew a relationship between us would never work. I felt complete and was ready to move on.

My not-yet-ex-husband knew William from church, could feel the energy between us, didn't want the divorce—or at least didn't want me to be with anyone else—and tried to scare William off by telling him that I was grossly disfigured from surgery and that I s--t in a bag. He also knew about my trip back to my hometown and told him I went there to sleep with some other guy. He didn't know I had already shared absolutely everything already with William as a friend.

WILLIAM

I thought *he's a crazy guy,* and I couldn't understand what difference it made that she had an ostomy. I have false teeth on top, and so what? I get emotional when I recall that time because I knew I loved Anita as soon as I saw her. I am a recovering alcoholic. I had been married three times before, and this was the first time I had ever gotten into a relationship while being sober. It felt spiritual to me in a way I had never experienced with anyone before.

ANITA

In the meantime, William's relationship with his fiancée was going downhill fast, the main issue being that she was becoming extremely religious in a way that wasn't at all comfortable for him. The more we talked and learned about each other, the more I realized this was the guy I was looking for. Falling in love with him made it harder and harder to keep on that friend hat. William and his fiancée finally broke up four months after we met, and our first date was five days later on Memorial Day weekend.

We had three dates in four days, and on the third date we were talking about the relationship in general and how amazing everything was. William said, "We are going to be getting married."

I was stunned and terrified even though I was hugely attracted to him and knew it was meant to be. I was also very clear with him, "I have been married to two angry, controlling men. I have a lot of healing to do, and it will have to happen in the context of this relationship. I want you to be aware of what you are signing up for with me."

We meditated together that week and went to another place or dimension where Spirit came down, surrounded us with light, put our hands together, and said, "The union of your souls has been blessed." We both absolutely trusted that.

We had been friends for four months, and as products of the seventies, it was new for both of us to have a strong foundation of friendship before intimacy. About a week after we had been officially dating, we were necking on the couch and I dragged him into the bedroom.

WILLIAM

I was very attracted to Anita from the first moment I saw her, and we made love many times in my imagination before we ever got together in person. Seeing the bag for the first time, I was surprised how small it was. I didn't really know anything about her stoma and asked if I could lie on top of her during intercourse without hurting it. She showed me the scar on her butt, and I thought it looked pretty neat. I had never seen a butt sewn shut before. I had experienced anal sex before and really enjoyed it, but I didn't feel sad that we would never be able to do that. It was only a little disappointing at the time, and I can't say I have missed it.

ANITA

When I had been so sick off and on with proctitis, the thought of anal sex scared me, and I never wanted anything near there. I had only tried it once. It was so painful that I never wanted to do it again, and I was very happy that now that door was now literally closed. I did feel self-conscious about the proctectomy scar, since it is bumpy and sticks out.

WILLIAM

It turned out that the scar she felt self-conscious about aided in my stimulation when we couldn't have regular intercourse and tried other positions; having the ostomy turned out to be a benefit in this case because the raised, bumpy ridge feels really good when I rub against it.

ANITA

Soon after we started dating and having sex we were taking a shower together. My bag was off and my ostomy did its thing—I pooped in the shower and I was mortified. William just laughed and took his foot and shoved it down the drain; it didn't bother him in the least.

WILLIAM

I didn't know the stoma was going to be so cute, it's just a nice little red thing sticking out. I like being around when Anita changes her bag so I can see it. I was mystified as to why she was so embarrassed since it's a natural thing. I especially like taking a shower with her on the mornings when she changes her bag because she takes off the old one first. After over four years together, I love seeing her stoma.

ANITA

The ostomy has *never* been a problem in our sex life, though there have actually been many other completely unrelated health issues that have all resulted in chronic vaginitis, which has very significantly affected it. We have found other ways to physically love each other beside intercourse when I am having problems, and I am extremely grateful for William's creativity, flexibility, and patience.

Not everybody is going to be William, and I am so glad I was able to move on to have this healthy, happy relationship. I worried for years about being rejected over my ostomy, but he has wholeheartedly accepted that part of me and it feels great.

Once we were in foreplay and he was kissing me all over, and I felt a pressure on my stoma. I didn't believe it at first, but I realized he was kissing it through the bag. It makes me cry now when I remember that because it felt like such a huge acknowledgement.

"Did you just kiss my stoma?"

He nodded.

"Why?"

"Because I love 100 percent of you."

—— ⊛ ——

SMILING—AT LAST!

LESLIE GILBERT-GRUNDER

I am a forty-nine-year-old woman who has three great kids, a husband, grandson, and a dog living together in our house with banging aluminum siding in the city of Philadelphia. We have our moments of chaos with us all laughing, hollering, and running around along with the family having calm times of doing homework and reading while they wait anxiously for dinner to be finished.

Life wasn't always fun for me. Diagnosed at age twenty-five with Crohn's disease, I remember suffering with bad belly behaviors since high school. The thing I feared the most was getting a colostomy bag. I cried, screamed, and even changed doctors and hospitals during flare-ups if anyone even mentioned going that route. It seemed a fate worse than death.

You would think after much pain, fistulas, dehydration, and constant diarrhea, I would be agreeable to an ostomy. Ironically, it wasn't until a hole was torn in my colon while removing a polyp that I was forced to have emergency surgery, and I woke up groggily hearing my mom ask the doctor if it could be reversed.

When I came home after surgery, I was stapled up and those staples dug into my skin. I couldn't distinguish the pain from the inside or the outside; I fell into a dark depression. I did nothing for a while but stare at the walls and silently cry. I felt ugly, gross, and embarrassed. I didn't want anyone near me. I tried not to eat or drink much so there would be less in the bag, but then I became dehydrated and light headed.

So much went through my head. I didn't want to feel like an old person before my time, and all I thought about was how disgusting I was. I tortured myself with things I was unable to do. I missed rubbing my hands along my belly to feel the soft, smooth skin there. Through talks with my husband, I started to see the colostomy bag differently. He showed me that it didn't matter to him and that helped me relax.

The good news is I am no longer depressed about the colostomy. I have learned to live with it. The fistulas went away, no more bowel movements coming out of my vagina, and I started to feel human again. Since having a colostomy, we have our sex life back, and I enjoy sex again now that my body has healed and I am no longer on medications. We are having the best time with exploring parts that haven't felt so alive in forever. My husband says I am making up for lost climaxing time. Orgasm after orgasm and they do feel great. I never knew what I was missing. I feel blessed to have a husband who finds me sexy regardless of the bag.

I had always been embarrassed about my body, even before the colostomy. I always thought I was too fat or saggy, and sometimes I look back at pictures of myself, remembering how horrible I felt about my body at the time, and I just sigh because now I see that I was pretty. I wish I would have known it then. It has only been a few years that I am able to accept myself as I am. I feel alive again and it shows by the smile on my face.

───── ⊛ ─────

THE FORTY-EIGHT-YEAR WAIT
CARLAND KERR

There were several reasons I waited until I was forty-eight years old to get married. With having an ostomy for twenty years, I learned how to pick out the mean guys pretty quickly. Usually around the third date I would let them know about the ostomy. I didn't want to get attached if they couldn't handle it, plus it revealed the true character of the guy.

Once after the show-and-tell, one guy couldn't get out of the house fast enough. Another compared my bag to the local paper saying, "I can't date someone who has the news journal hanging from them."

They weren't all bad. I went out with another guy for a long time, but we split for reasons that had nothing to do with having an ostomy.

Bill was different. I took a four-year break before I met him. We met online and chatted a month back and forth before we even talked on the phone. We took it slow by asking each other two online questions per e-mail. I was glad he was never inappropriate with asking sexual questions.

Then we moved to the telephone, and finally went on our first date to Chili's, followed by a date playing pool. On the third date, we were in my house when I knew it was time to broach the subject. I liked him but didn't want to be emotionally invested if it couldn't go anywhere.

We were sitting on the sofa, and I was nervously fidgeting and trying to tell him. "I have something to tell you … it's nothing you can catch. When I was eighteen, I was diagnosed with Crohn's disease. Do you know what that is?"

"No," he said hesitantly.

"I'll explain it later. I got really sick and then I had to have surgery. Um, ah, um," I kept delaying the inevitable. Finally I stood up because I was nervous and didn't intend to show him my bag, but as I stood up, my shorts fell to my hips. I didn't realize how loose they were. "Well, here I have a bag." I pointed to it.

He seemed a little surprised, "Oh, okay, that's all right, that doesn't change you or what I think about you."

Date five was at my house. We didn't plan anything; it just kind of happened. I always wear a short nightgown to cover my bag. He lifted my nightgown and never said anything—it was never an issue.

He's cool about it and doesn't tell people or broadcast it. He's always worried about me getting sick and he's very protective. I waited forty-eight years to get married, and he's the greatest.

LOOK FORWARD—SOMETHING AWAITS
CHARLOTTE TAYLOR

At age seventeen I had an ostomy reversal after my colon healed from colon cancer. Later I found out my family had a 100 percent chance of having colon cancer. I was diagnosed with FAP (Familial Adenomatous Polyposis), an inherited colorectal cancer syndrome with the onset of the rare Gardner's syndrome, where polyps grow randomly outside of the colon. In the generation just before me, my generation, and the one after me, there were nine of us with an ostomy, J-pouch, or Koch pouch. It's so prevalent that our family is registered in the Cleveland Clinic.

I got married in 1970, and four years later I had to have ileostomy surgery; polyps were growing faster than they could be removed. After the surgery, I woke up to my husband standing by my bed. He was looking at the pouch I had on and said "I have never seen anything so fascinating."

We never had a problem with it. I wore pouch covers and he was there for me. One time at a challenging time in our marriage when I found out he had an affair, I was hurt and said to him, "What does she have that I don't have? Oh, I know—I have a pouch and she doesn't!"

Immediately he responded, "Don't ever blame yourself for having an ileostomy because it's nothing to be ashamed about. I never want you to think that again."

It took a while to get over it, but we had thirty-nine wonderful years before he passed away. You can make your ostomy whatever you want it to be. I've lived a wonderful life and each day is a blessing; it is also what you make it. When I go out and someone asks me how I am, I always respond with, "I am blessed."

I'm a survivor of cancer and the tornado that hit Huntsville, Alabama, November 15, 1989, which totaled my car with me inside it. I looked up and the tornado was coming at me. All the windows exploded in the car and the tires ripped off the rims. I was still in the car when it was over, but the only thing I can remember was that I was praying in the name of Jesus. My car was lifted, and I ended up in front of the First National Bank. I didn't pass out, but I fell over in the seat and threw one hand over my head. My body was full of slivers of glass. They used masking tape to pull it out. I had my ostomy at that time, and I automatically threw my other hand over my stomach to protect it. My hand was hurt, I had nightmares for a while, and every time it was windy, I got a little nervous. Over time the anxiety lessened.

Now that my husband is gone, I think back on things he said to me. Whenever I wore my swim suit or dress pants, he always said I looked nice in my clothes. I never had a problem talking about the ostomy to anyone. I do feel a little funny now that I am single, and I'm still young enough to think about marriage again. One thing that always impressed my husband was the fact that I didn't let my ileostomy stand in the way of our intimacy.

I enjoy looking on the websites and there is a gentleman from Kansas City who has an ostomy, and I thought I might like to meet him. I don't spend a lot of time chatting online but it's good for information. It's good to be able to contact people through the Internet. I am sixty-six years old and grateful for every day. I miss my husband. He had a small stroke that preceded a massive stroke and then was paralyzed and blind and lived for another seven months. I was never unfaithful to him, but I am still young enough to think about a new relationship. I look forward to it.

—— ⚘ ——

DOING IS BETTER THAN FEARING
CHERYL CLEVELAND

I was told I was the youngest person in Tennessee to receive an ileostomy due to ulcerative colitis. I was age seventeen at that time. It was hard to have an ileostomy and in some ways it was a huge blessing. It was my senior year of school, and I was focused on getting out of the hospital to graduate and be with my friends. I had a boyfriend already and had been sexually active with him before and after surgery.

I didn't have self-esteem issues until I was twenty-two when I was thrown back into the dating world. *How am I going to tell people I have this?* It was a constant worry. I never had any intimacy challenges with people, probably because I got to know them a little bit before I got into that situation with them.

In several of my relationships I must have prolonged having sex too long. I would wait until we were having dinner and drinks and then I went into detail about having had a disease and then I'd finally admit I had an ileostomy. I would do this big build-up and most people told me something like, "Oh, okay, I thought you were going to tell me you were gay."

I was single for eleven years after having been married for a while; the ostomy was never an issue.

I met my husband on a Friday, and it was love at first sight. My husband and I slept together three days after I met him—he was persistent. We were in the kitchen cooking dinner and about to have steaks.

"I am very attracted to you, why don't we forget dinner and move on upstairs?" he asked.

"There's something I have to tell you, I was sick when I was seventeen and had to have a bag on my stomach as the result of surgery," I offered.

"Like a plastic bag? A baggie? Let me see it," he said.

I unzipped my jeans.

He looked at me, "Let's go upstairs."

I learned early on not to get into a huge medical explanation; it's too much information. Intimacy has been great, and we've only had two situations where my bag (named Fred) came off. My husband said, "I feel something. Oh my gosh, Fred has come off!"

I remember I was embarrassed. My husband was on top, there was a lot of friction, and maybe I didn't have the snap on well. He jumped out of bed, "Let me get something to clean it up." We got in the shower, cleaned it up, and went back to what we were doing. I have never been uncomfortable or felt like I needed an ostomy cover.

Everyone gives advice on how long to wait and how you should tell people. I didn't tell one guy for six weeks. I think I just knew. It depends on how you present it to the person you are telling. If you are like *oh my God, this is horrible, I hope you accept me*, it won't go over so well. If you present it like *this is me and this happened and accept me for who I am*, it should work out.

I am now a fifty-five-year-old mother of a seven-year-old adopted child and have been married twenty years. When I got out of the hospital, I heard all these rules—don't drive, don't eat popcorn, don't have sex, don't water ski, don't, don't, don't! I was home a week and had done everything except water ski, but I never did that anyway. We can live under the fear of don'ts or start doing today—and doing is much better.

———— ✤ ————

INTIMATE OPTIONS
Donna Lemison

My boyfriend is blind in one eye and deaf. We met in a program for veterans struggling with post-traumatic stress disorder (PTSD). I liked him immediately when I saw him. He's ten years older than I am, and we are both ex-military. I asked him to the Marine Ball, and we started dating after that.

I got my ostomy in July 2010, after suffering for six years with impacted bowels and severe constipation. It was an elected surgery, but I have no regrets. My kids thought I was crazy to be willing to have a bag attached to me for the rest of my life, but I couldn't stand the constipation pain that could last for a week and then the trauma of the bowel movement. I am only fifty-one, but this bag is now a part of me.

My boyfriend can't have sex, and we are intimate by touching and feeling each other. I thought having the ostomy was going to be ugly, but he doesn't mind touching my body and the bag. He loves to kiss me and hug me. We do all the normal things people do in having sex except intercourse. I've never had anybody treat me the way he does in love-making. He has taken a real interest in me and my body and views me as a person instead of a sex object.

With other men, sex was approached like, *Let's get it over with*, and it was always about the guy's pleasure and never anything with me. My boyfriend treats me totally different, and he thinks I am beautiful, even with the ostomy. We are going on eighteen months and are still relatively new in our relationship. He could have said no thanks to the ostomy and walked away, but he didn't.

When I received the ostomy, my boyfriend tried to learn everything he could about it, including trying to put it on me. In doing the wafer, he measured the inches. He wanted to know each detail about the ostomy and how it worked. He said to me, "If you are going through this, I am going through this with you." He really tried to understand what it was like for me to have the bag hanging off of me. Even though we have an unusual sex life, he is tender, gentle, caring, and loving. He took an interest in everything.

Another life-saver for me was some products I ordered online. I especially like the micro-fiber piece of material that goes around the whole body that holds the ostomy in place. The panties I bought and the swimwear brought me back to a normalcy in life. They make me feel better about myself.

Even though my boyfriend and I are only intimate by touching, that's our sex life. A good sex life is when both of you participate and both of you are pleasured, and ours qualifies.

---— ⟨ℬ⟩ ———

ACCEPTANCE AND TRUST
Doug Marchant

I got served divorce papers while I was in the hospital having ileostomy surgery for the Crohn's disease that had torn through my intestines and caused peritonitis. I was so sick, I died three times. While I was in the hospital for a seven-month stretch to save my life, the divorce papers were actually a favor done for me. I had no intention of going back to my three-year turbulent marriage.

Diagnosed with Crohn's disease when I was twenty-six, I had my first surgery within a year. Prior to that time I went through the usual questioning about stress, nerves, as if it was all in my head. When you find out you have Crohn's disease, it's really bittersweet. You can't get rid of the disease but at last you have a diagnosis that's in black and white. I could finally understand why my body was kicking my own butt. Finally, I could look at people and say, it's not in my head, it's real—like the old story with the guy whose tombstone read, "I told you I was sick!"

Recuperation took a long time from my surgeries. I was bordering on some serious depression and drinking too much. I was a mess. I remember talking to the doctor about my concerns for intimacy. I was afraid I was going to hurt myself physically after all I had gone through. He said something that stuck with me forever, "If two porcupines can do it without killing each other, I think you'll be just fine." That helped lessen my worries.

It was five years before I met my second wife (now married for fifteen years), and she was my life saver. If she hadn't come along, I probably would have killed myself. She pulled me out of the gutter, and I pulled her out of her abusive marriage.

Two years ago I had to have everything moved from one side to another, a stoma revision. The nurses asked my wife if she could take on the role of changing the dressing. The visiting nurses taught her about the wound care. Even though we'd been together for thirteen years, I felt exposed having my wife caring for me like this. You can't feel more naked than when you are laying there with a massive open wound and your loved one has to help you. It's not a good naked either; you are at your most vulnerable. With so many operations over the years, I've been carved more than a Thanksgiving turkey.

If a person with an ostomy is planning on being intimate with someone and has too much anxiety, my view is either you don't trust that person enough or perhaps you are still having trouble accepting the ostomy yourself. The good thing for me is that I don't plan on having an end to my story or sex life until I am too old to walk. Even then, who knows?

—— ✿ ——

LIVE AND LOVE
George Salamy

I learned early on that if I could accept my ostomy, my partner would be okay with it, too. Five years into my marriage with Barbara, I was too sick with ulcerative colitis, and an ileostomy became necessary. I already had one child and more on the way. With surgery, doctors don't guarantee anything. Most likely I'd be fine, but one never knows.

I was in a Manhattan, New York, hospital for two weeks. My wife worked for the president of New York medical college and the chief of pediatrics at this hospital. She later became a nurse. On the way up to see me on my last night in the hospital, she stopped at a kiosk at the subway and bought a dirty magazine for me. I called her later that night and told her everything was working. I was glad they didn't have to cut that deeply—my surgery was standard.

After the first couple of weeks, I didn't want to do anything. I was wearing the clear pouches as well as the vinyl pouches that one rinsed off, and I wasn't sure how it was going to work. After surgery, it took me a couple of months to get things squared away, to get healthy again.

I went back to work part-time. Then one night we declared, "Tonight's the night!" We gave it a shot, and it kept working. After a while, I taped the pouch up to get it out of the way so it wasn't hanging down and catching on anything.

Ironically, Barbara was diagnosed with ovarian cancer and eventually ended up with a temporary ileostomy. Her belly was distended because of the disease and the placement of the stoma made it difficult for her to handle the pouch. She needed help getting the pouch on two to three times a week, and I helped her change it. She was a caregiver for me, and I felt good to do it in return. For thirty years we had an enviable marriage. Sadly, Barbara died of ovarian cancer.

Almost four years later, I married again. One year after Barbara died I had a time frame in my head about moving forward. After almost a year, I met a woman who knew my wife. We met serendipitously at a mutual friend's birthday party. Linda had been widowed for nine years. I ran into her and asked her how she was doing. Our chemistry clicked right away. She still had a daughter in school and another marriage was not in the cards for her for a little while. Her other daughter was getting married, and my daughter had just gotten married. We waited for our kids to get their big events over, like finishing up school and getting a job. She was a school teacher, and we dated for three years. Once our kids were somewhat set, things were a little more settled.

After we dated for three years, she decided to retire. She questioned, "What's going on and where are we going with this?"

I wasn't ready yet. I was trying to manage the grief period my kids were going through. The grief of a spouse is different for the children. I can have another woman in my life, but they will never have another mother. They wanted me to date rather than get serious with one, and it took awhile before the timing was right.

Early into the relationship, about six months, I wanted her to know I had an ileostomy. I told her I had been sick, had surgery, and then I gave her a book from the UOAA, a guide book on ileostomies—they have them available on all the surgeries. "I am going to leave this with you. I want you to read this thing. If you have a problem with this, then we have a problem."

She read the guide and had no problem with it. She was a little surprised and said it didn't bother her, and later she said, "You never complain about it."

"What's there to complain about?" I asked

Linda just took it in stride.

Finally the time came to try things out. It wasn't the best sex at first because neither of us had been sexual for a while, but soon, after we figured it all out. It worked fine. We were both so nervous, but it didn't take long for everything to cooperate. Linda never commented about my pouch, and she adjusted to it beautifully.

Many people in general stay in relationships because they don't know what it will be like to go out on the market with an ostomy. When I was ready to move forward, I thought *I have to deal with this*. If someone was uncomfortable and couldn't handle it, I told myself I'd say, "Have a nice day. Next?"

I am sure there are people that are so secretive about it and all of a sudden if they have to go out to meet someone, they might panic. I knew I would be involved with another woman and get married somehow—it was in my DNA. You have to be comfortable in your skin, and I was confident in myself. If you are worried about odor and this and that, it's never going to happen.

I was so young when I got sick, drug options were limited. These days, they medicate you to death. The surgery was the best thing I ever did. I could eat and not have to worry anymore. I traveled around the world for my job, extensively to Asia, and that would never have happened if I didn't have the surgery. An ostomy was even better in some places because I didn't have to worry about the bathrooms.

I participated as a rider in the Get Your Guts In Gear bike ride a couple of times and played racquetball for years after surgery. I golf, swim, and am in the gym three or four mornings a week on the bike, treadmill, and lifting weights. It feels good to be alive and have someone to love again.

———— ⊛ ————

I DREAMED HER TO LIFE
GORDON MANEY

I discovered the love of my life on the Internet when I first read Carol's profile and looked at her pictures. Who can explain what is appealing, other than an indefinable constellation of points to which we respond? Appealing comes from the facts and ideas, how they are presented, and what they seem to reveal about the person. Her profile was nicely written. She liked big dogs and scuba diving. My favorite picture was one of her in a patchwork sweater. I found her to be very interesting. And really cute.

Over a period of days I came back and looked at Carol's photograph many times. Finally I worked up the courage to send her a note.

"My favorite picture of you is the one in the patchwork sweater."

That was the entire note. Would I ever hear from her? Days passed. I guessed not. Then a reply!

We began sending little notes back and forth. They became longer and deeper, more interesting and meaningful. The heart and mind of a woman was being revealed to me. I wanted to learn more.

After some correspondence over a period of weeks, struggling with my impatience to meet her, I asked Carol if she wanted to telephone me as a transitional step to the possibility of meeting in person. I had already told her the URL for my website, given her my home address, and my home and cell phone numbers—all to assure her I was trustworthy. I even told her I was not an axe murderer. She thanked me for that assurance, saying it eased her mind immensely.

Carol said *yes*, she would phone me.

I wanted to be very careful because I felt I was nurturing the delicate possibility of a beautiful future, and I was also extremely excited to meet her in person. She phoned; we had a wonderful conversation that flowed easily. I believed it was illuminating with respect to possibilities. We each wanted to meet, that was quite apparent.

I dressed nervously for our first meeting. Was it a date? I did not know, but it certainly felt very important. I arrived at the restaurant early, to be sure not to be late. I spent some minutes analyzing where to sit as I waited. Should I appear relaxed? Should I appear alert? How should I sit? As if all that would make *any* difference at all.

A black car drove by the window as I sat on a bench in the lobby. I strained to see into the car's window, wondering if it was the woman in the patchwork sweater. Minutes later the restaurant door opened. A smiling woman came inside and stopped at the bench where I was sitting.

"I'm Carol," she said, holding her hand out to me.

She charmed me in that moment. She has not stopped charming me since. Her look, her voice, her smile, and her way. I call it the *Carol way*.

We were seated in the restaurant and fell immediately into happy talk, unaware of the waitress waiting to take our order. We laughed when we noticed her, quickly ordered, and then continued our exchange. It was the kind of quickly moving conversation shared by two people excited to be in one another's presence. I remember most of all that it was really wonderful, and I did not want it to end.

Not long after we were engaged in conversation, I took her hands in mine. In that moment I reflected on the notion that to do so could seem bold. Yet it seemed right to me, and Carol's hands did so invite me. I was lost in her smile, the sound of her voice, and the feel of her hands in mine. We had a really nice time that evening. I did not want to leave her.

Because I was liking her so much, I reached a point where I asked if we could meet again the following Monday. Carol said she could not, because she had an ostomy support meeting.

"What is the meaning of ostomy?" I asked her.

I was somewhat familiar with the term colostomy, yet in that moment I really did not grasp the link between ostomy and colostomy. I knew there were people who pooped in a bag, yet I had never seen such a bag. I knew a woman who did that, but she never talked about it.

Carol described a bit about her history, and I got a detailed explanation of how the end of the intestine is formed into a stoma. I had to imagine all that since I had never seen one before.

I later learned she was certain I had Googled her and learned of her ostomy support group involvement, with the obvious implications. I had not. I had spent my time admiring her in that patchwork sweater.

"I don't care…." were the very next words out of my mouth.

Carol was far too interesting and appealing to have that make any difference to me. Years ago I would have cared. I would not have been able to imagine being with someone who pooped in a bag. I don't think I could have coped with me pooping in a bag. In fact, I'm sure of it.

I had, however, new perspectives from my own medical experiences. I found them as I fearfully watched ceiling tile go by overhead one day, on the way to a cath lab. I found them while lying in a cold room, connected to wires, hearing beeps coincide exactly with the pounding upheaval in my chest. I found them while viewing again a bright sun and a clear sky when I returned to the world outdoors.

I understood, wordlessly, that Carol knew things others did not. I knew she had new perspectives, as I did. She understood more than most about what is truly important.

All that made her more appealing to me. In this moment, as I write this, I realize Carol is more appealing to me because she has an ostomy. Her imperfection—her experience—makes her more perfect in her appeal. This difference in her makes her even more beautiful to me.

We concluded our second date at the restaurant. What I knew most of all from that meeting was that I wanted to see Carol again, and very soon. She said she would like that, too. I walked Carol to her car, not wanting to leave her presence. I asked her if she would like a hug, nervously awaiting an answer. She said yes, with a smile, and wrapped her arms around me. It was wonderful. I did not kiss her because I was trying to be careful. I had an ever-growing sense of the possibilities.

We met again, had a wonderful time, and dated more and more. Mutual appeal and affection grew. She invited me to her house to meet her dogs. That seems a small thing, but dog people know it is not. I received introductions to her dogs, Jack and Sydney, just as one might for people. We did a lot of ear scratching, petting, and dog talk as Jack and Sydney jockeyed for position to see which could get more attention. There was much tail wagging. I had passed a crucial test. That, along with the fact that I own a one-hundred-pound Alaskan Malamute, verified my canine compatibility.

After a time of growing closer together, we both instinctively and word-lessly knew we would become sexually intimate. I was confident Carol's ostomy would not matter to me. I was concerned that Carol may have been worried about how I would respond. I believed that once we made love, she would know it did not matter to me.

We did talk of sexual intimacy before we experienced it. We talked about the bag and whether it would move around. I wanted to learn all I could to engage with Carol in such a way that she was not self-conscious and also cause her to know in her heart that I found her extremely desirable.

"What do I need to know?" I asked. "Do I need to be careful in some way?"

I have had my own medical issues. I have had cardiac ablations to correct two separate heart rhythm problems, and I had one testicle removed, so I elected to write something I could read to Carol. It was, in essence, an inventory of what all is wrong with me. I remember crying as I wrote it for her and crying as I read it to her. Not because of how I felt about me, but because I cared so much for her and wanted to reach her emotionally so she could feel safe.

I can only try to imagine what it would be like to have an ostomy and wonder how I might be regarded in a sexually intimate situation with some-one new. I might fear the bag would be all the other person could see. My reality was that all I could see was Carol. I did not notice the bag at all.

We made love that first time; yet another new and very important way to meet. It was beautiful, glorious, warm, and human. No bag was present, only the two of us. The only thing between us was our shared, passionate connection. I tell Carol I dreamed her to life. The origin of that expression— *I dreamed you to life*—is a song by the group Savage Garden.

Life is earthy, gritty, and sometimes uncomfortably real. One cannot hide from these realities and still live fully, honestly, and happily. Having an ostomy brings the gritty side of life out in the open—quite regularly, as osto-mates know all too well. In that sense, people who seem perfect in form are at a disadvantage. They may hide from reality and be easily frightened by it.

"Things don't have to be perfect to be perfect," Carol said to me once. That statement applies to ostomates.

Standing in the shower one day, drying myself with a towel, I watched Carol at the sink, changing her bag. I laughed as I looked down at the floor and saw poop on the tile. My first thought? *I love this little woman.*

Carol runs a local ostomy support group. I participate regularly and with enthusiasm. We also attend regional meetings and events pertaining to ostomates and inflammatory bowel diseases. We discuss issues of importance to ostomates. I find satisfaction in helping others by sharing my perspectives as a support person. I understand much about their lives from living with Carol. You see, I have new perspectives.

I help Carol change her bag and attend to those occasional emergencies that inevitably occur. We laugh together as I hand her the wipes or clean the floor. We are partners in everything. The fact that Carol has an ostomy makes her no less appealing to me—physically, sexually, mentally, or emotionally. Quite the opposite. I find her beautiful, charming, and desirable in all the ways important for companionship, relationship, sexual intimacy, and marriage. I dreamed her to life. She is my queen.

———— ✆ ————

LOVE IS MORE THAN SEX
Judy Tipton

Because of the Agent Orange my husband was exposed to in Vietnam, he developed a tumor, B-cell non-Hodgkin lymphoma, in his tailbone. He also has diabetes, which gives him neuropathy in his hands and feet. He's numb all the way around from his waist to his back from surgery and has a constant pain where his tailbone used to be.

During surgery in 2004, they cut his bladder and bowel nerves. That pretty much ended our love life. We can't have sex; he's got a bladder tube in his penis that goes down into a leg bag. He didn't want to even touch me anymore because he was afraid he'd get me excited and he couldn't do anything about it.

We were very sexually active and romantic before this happened, even though we have been married thirty-four years now. When he comes in the house to this day, my heart still flutters. I missed the hugging and the loving he used to give me. He knew I missed it. Once in a while I would ask him why he couldn't hold me anymore.

He would say, "You know I love you."

I'd say, "Sometimes, I just want to be hugged and kissed even though I know you love me."

The surgery changed his physical reaction where he could not get aroused anymore. He doesn't even say he misses it. I suggested we go to a sex store to see if there was something we could use to get him excited and he wasn't interested in that either—doesn't believe in that kind of thing. I loved him and he didn't hold me, touch me, or do anything romantic anymore. It broke my heart. He used to rub my feet. He's always been a quiet man, but I like to talk and I am a talker.

He's got a sad medical situation, but I have loved him from hello. He has a colostomy and he deals with it. I have to put the flange on him because he can't do that part very well, but that's only once or twice a week. He went into a diabetic coma and his fingers didn't come out of it working right. He has limited use, but he can change his pouch daily on his own.

One day not too long ago he had a PTSD (post-traumatic stress disorder) episode and he really scared me. I didn't feel like going to church in the morning because I knew I couldn't get ready in time because of my arm. I wanted to go that night. He got that devil look in his face. A woman knows when something's going to happen. He had an attitude that morning when he went to church, and I had a sick feeling in my stomach. He got mad and snapped big time. I was afraid he was going to hurt me. My first husband used to beat me all the time, and I have a fear of that. It never leaves you.

He had never used that kind of profanity against me, and he never talked like that. His eyes were wild looking, and then he sped off in the truck. My daughter followed him in her vehicle. He noticed her and eventually pulled over and then he calmed down. My daughter told him, "You need to go home to Momma; she's scared."

When he got home, I said, "You are going to the doctor tomorrow and you are going on medication because you frightened me. I didn't know if you were going to hurt me, but I knew it wasn't good."

The next day the doctor put him on an anti-depressant and within a week I could tell the difference.

It shocked me when one day he walked right up behind me and hugged me. He used to give me a tiny peck and now he gives me a good kiss on the lips. He does more for me now, folding the laundry, and anything I want, he'll buy it for me. It's a big change and a welcome one. He started showing me how much he loved me again.

I just had rotator cuff surgery, and he shows his love for me in many other ways besides sex. He helps me around the house and takes care of me when I am sick. That's marriage—even if you can't have sex, you can be romantic, love each other, and kiss. The sexual part doesn't matter; if they hug you and give you some attention, that's all you need.

———— ✦ ————

SELF-INTIMACY
LOUISE (ANONYMOUS)

I am a lesbian, and I haven't (by choice) had a woman in my life for many years. I am afraid to become sexually involved since my ostomy surgery and even saying I am a lesbian is still new to me. I have never admitted it to anyone but my daughters.

Since my ostomy surgery one year ago for colorectal cancer, I haven't been with a male or female, and I don't know if I ever will again. The thought of a partner seeing me with my pouch is very difficult. Although one good thing about having the cancer is that it allowed me to say, "This is who I am. Take me or leave me."

I have not made any efforts to have a relationship with anyone, and I asked my One Source (God), *If you want me to have someone in my life, bring them to me because I am not seeking it.*

It might be easier for me to meet someone with an ostomy like I have.

I'm not depressed; I just have not dealt with someone else accepting me with my body the way it is now. Instead, I have accepted being without a partner for now. I was raised under a very religious background with a big family, and I am becoming more open to saying yes if asked, "Are you a lesbian?"

But I am sure many would be shocked. I would be the last person they would expect to be a lesbian. I knew from the time I was a little girl, I loved the way girls looked, and I was fascinated by them and it never changed as I became a woman. With my strict religious upbringing, I suppressed those feelings and only had men in my life but never felt right. In fact, I had a very hard time throughout the eight years of marriage convincing myself that I had done the right thing.

I have only had one woman in my life. We had a nice relationship for a short while and so long ago that I have since lost contact.

The only person I have a sexual relationship with these days is me. While I masturbate, I am not as horny as I used to be. I am not sure if it's because of the ostomy, but even when I touch myself, I find I want to cover the bag—it's too distracting for even me.

I haven't had a good session in a long time. Since the ostomy, I have had shorter sessions. I want to be free with myself. I hope that eventually I'll get over the need to cover my bag when I am playing with myself. As far as feeling sexy, I have not felt great about myself for a while—maybe I just need a new toy or something. It probably has something to do with self-image.

I truly love myself. I couldn't always say that. I was born with club feet and that was difficult, too. I love myself now, but there are areas of how I look that I still don't like, and maybe the crackling sound of the pouch bothers me, too. I have a good life with my grown children and grandchildren. We'll see what my One Source has in store for me.

———— ✥ ————

TWO LIVES, TWO HEARTS, TOGETHER AS ONE
NANCY AND GARY CHOW

NANCY

My husband, Gary, and I both lost our previous spouses to cancer. We had both tried dating and nothing seemed to work out until we met each other on eHarmony.com. I met Gary eight months after my husband passed away at age fifty-eight of prostate cancer.

Prior to meeting Gary, I had one date that showed promise. I said, "Before anything happens here, I have something to tell you. I have had Crohn's disease for thirty years, and now I have an ileostomy and wear a bag. I have never had a symptom since."

He looked at me like I told him the worst thing in the world. All he could say was, "I don't know how that's going to affect the sex life." We quickly went our separate ways.

On my first date with Gary, we talked a little bit about our histories. On the second date, we ended up across the street from where my first husband had worked. It was there I told Gary that I had major surgery seven years earlier.

He asked, "Do you mind if I ask what the major surgery was?"

I told him, "I had Crohn's disease, and I have an ileostomy," and then explained details further. I asked him, "Is that a problem for you?"

He was quick to answer, "Why would it be?"

Wow, I thought. It was wonderful that someone I just met for the second time was so accepting of it, and I became more attracted to him. On our first Valentine's Day, we went out for a romantic dinner and came back to Gary's house, and I spent the night. We were snuggled up in each other's arms when I woke up and you-know-what was everywhere, and I was mortified.

"Nancy, don't worry about it. You get in the shower, and I'll clean up the bedding."

I had a major blow out and he dealt with it. I took a shower and went to work the next day and said to my coworkers, "You're never going to believe this." I told them about my accident and what I had said to Gary. "I should be cleaning up after myself. This is my problem."

He said, "Nancy, this is our problem. Would you mind if I watch when you change your ostomy? I would like to know how to change it if you ever need me to."

GARY

Nancy can take care of herself, but she knows I'll be there to help her if she's unable to. I would always step in if she couldn't. Since I took care of my wife with cancer, you learn. It's all part of loving a person. Sometimes people get frustrated—we all do. Step back, look at things, and jump on the horse again to make it work. I am here to be her cheerleader and to help her cope with any situations as she does with me. Because I work for the American Cancer Society, I have worked with ostomates before, although I've never been intimate with anyone that had one. But they are people like anyone else. You are going to have s--t one way or another, whether it's in the bag or in the bowl. We both had twenty-five years of good marriages. When you meet someone new, it's part of the whole package you go in with. There were other qualities I was looking at to see if Nancy was the right person for me and having an ostomy was not something I would judge a person on.

I was looking for a woman who could take my shortcomings and, in spite of them, want to stick around with me. I hoped she would enjoy the things I do and allow me to experience her world also and we both grow from enjoying those personal experiences. We both had our issues. Many a woman has turned me down, too. Would Nancy be willing to stick around and enjoy someone like me with my kind of baggage?

When the accident happened with Nancy, well, neither of us are exactly thrilled to have s--t all over the place. It's not exactly appetizing, but you have to consider your partner and realize the embarrassment she is going through. The biggest challenge when people are dating is the tendency to look for the prince charming, the princess, or the playmate of the month. When you've been around the block like we have, you look for other things that are more important in life. The qualities Nancy has were much more worth it than the extra kind of baggage she brings. Besides, if you have lived at all, everyone brings baggage to the relationship. How you use the baggage determines the success of the relationship.

NANCY

Once we were necking and the ileostomy was farting. I was afraid Gary would be turned off. Later he called me and said, "Don't worry about it because now I can fart in front of you."

I am required to take continuing education classes as a nurse and a couple of months after we met, I had gone to a class about taking care of ostomies as a nurse. I realized this was something I was really interested in. It would require me to get my bachelor's degree and then some specialized further training at Emory University. Gary had gone with me to WOC Nurse and UOAA conferences, and he supported me every step along the way. We were separated when I was in Atlanta attending school, and he flew out every three weeks. He's the love of my life, and I couldn't ask for anyone better because he's perfect for me.

GARY

You know that old saying, "If life gives you lemons, you make lemonade." When I lost my wife to cancer, I learned to use that unfortunate experience as a way to help other people who are going through the same things. With Nancy's nursing background, becoming a WOC Nurse was a no brainer. Taking her personal experience and her nursing skills into consideration, Emory recognized her potential and kept a position open for her at the school until she was able to attend.

NANCY

I always shared with patients that I had an ostomy even before as a staff nurse. If the patients were going to have an ostomy, I would introduce myself and tell them I had one and I'd like to help them with theirs. It's served the patients well to see someone that had a life and profession. When I was on the dating scene, it was helpful for them to know there were people out there who would be accepting. Even with the ostomy, our love life has been fabulous. Gary is a caring, gentle, considerate lover, and makes me feel like the most beautiful woman in the world even though I'm overweight and have a bag on my side—I am blessed.

GARY

Until my first wife passed away, she had been my only intimate contact with a woman. It was an education to date again, and you wonder how it is on the other side of the bedroom. Until you do it, you don't know what's out there. Of course, though, you still need to have the chemistry. If you find the right person and you can be sensitive to her needs, all will be well.

Nancy is the most passionate, loving, and perhaps the horniest woman I've ever met. She's forgiving of my problems, too. When she told me she had a bag, I told her I had ED (erectile dysfunction). If you feel there is a person that's special, you want to be as open as possible. You don't want to scare them away, but you want to see if a relationship can work out. That was part of our process of getting to know one another. Some women wouldn't be as patient with me. Nancy worked with me, was understanding, and we both had positive experiences even though it might not be conventional. It worked and if it works, run with it.

NANCY

For my final assignment at Emory, I was asked to write and present an in-service lecture. Mine was, "How to Put the O Back in Ostomy: Sex and the Ostomate."

We had discussions in class about dating and how to tell someone. There is a model that gives you the information as a WOC Nurse and how to bring up the subject. It should always be approached with the patients to allow them to bring up any issues about their sexuality. They need to know that if someone doesn't accept it, it's not the patient's fault. I talked about the intimate underwear available for people with ostomies, the different ways to make love; using vibrators; conventional sex; oral sex; gay, straight, transgender sex; and issues the patient had with having the rectum removed. Discussing these sometimes awkward issues that can affect sexuality is a vital part of obtaining the patient's informed consent.

The most important thing is to use your biggest sex organ, which is your mind, and if you use it right, everything else will follow. Basically, it's what you think about, your feelings, your consideration; it doesn't matter if you are gay or straight, female or male. Look at the person and give—if you give out, you're going to get back. We figure out what's going to make our partner feel good and when you can do that, things begin to move.

Sometimes people go into this as a contest. It's the wrong approach, as if who can get off faster is the most important thing in the relationship. So many people are used to "wham-bam-thank-you-ma'am." Many people don't understand that making love is not about just having sex, and if you truly make love, the sex can be fantastic. You do the normal touching but sometimes, depending on how a person reacts to your touch, you find you have to modify that and be patient. Sometimes a man may have a difficult time getting it up, some may need a lighter or heavier touch. Maybe they need lubrication or perhaps there are emotional issues involved. If you look for the great lovers in history—Valentino, Don Juan—they knew how to read a woman, to listen, to be sensitive, and I think that's the real secret to having a great relationship—be a little bit more liberal in how you approach it. Think out of the box.

Sometimes what works is not what you expected. Sex is not just about having an orgasm; it's a much bigger issue than that. It's all about making love.

Gary

I think that no man is an island. Couples have a lot of different resources at their disposal to enhance their relationship. Everyone has access to them if they open their eyes and talk and share. I have helped Nancy learn about things in regards to sex and there are a lot of organizations—UOAA, medical institutions, the American Cancer Society—that have great resources people should take advantage of. There are a lot of good counselors who can work with them if they are willing to go out there and grab the resources.

Many people have trouble listening to their partner. As Nancy has said, "God wants you to listen, that's why he gave you one mouth but two ears." Relationships are often treated like it's a final destination. It's the journey with your partner that counts.

Nancy

Love and understanding are the two most important things in giving. I want to please Gary as much as I can, and he gets joy in pleasing me as well. We got married in July 2008, and know we have an everlasting love.

——— ⊛ ———

YOU CAN GET YOUR LIFE BACK
Sarah Biggart

My husband and I were married in 1999. I got ulcerative colitis in the beginning of 2000. He likes to tease me saying he should have claimed the lemon law because I was defective. I was sick for five years and in that time, I got pregnant, lost my mother, and was really sick with ulcerative colitis. My son was only eighteen months old when it was determined I needed to have surgery.

Originally, the plan was for me to have a J-pouch, but it wasn't possible once they opened me up and saw the situation. The doctors came to tell my anxious family in the waiting room that they had to create an ostomy. I knew there was that possibility when I entered surgery. I was pretty groggy and on pain medicine when I woke up in the recovery room with my husband at my bedside. The first thing I asked him was, "Do I have a bag?"

My husband is a man of few words, "Yeah, they had to do it."

Later, my husband admitted how awful that moment was for him and how difficult it was to have to be the one to tell me. It was a moment that stays stuck in his mind.

I had been so sick with ulcerative colitis that on an average day I would be going to the bathroom forty-five times in a day, with constant diarrhea for five years. Luckily for me, I worked at home where we live and care for adults with disabilities. I don't think I would have been able to have any other kind of job.

As I lay there in the hospital bed, I noticed I was just lying there and not running to the toilet. That pastime consumed me every minute of every day.

I didn't have a problem accepting my ostomy because my ostomy gave me my life back. Once I had the ostomy, I could do all those things again. Even though I never would have wished this on myself, my life is so much better now. I can finally be the mom and wife I want to be. I can do things that were not an option before, like going to Disneyland. For the first time in years I can stand in line. Having the surgery was the right decision even though things didn't go smoothly. I had to make another trip to the ER because of a staph infection and abscess in my incision.

It was probably two months after surgery when I felt I should approach the subject of intimacy. In a matter-of-fact tone I said to my husband, "I feel like I'm ready and when you are ready, I am ready." I put the ball in his court. I'm a self-confident person. I felt okay with the bag, but I didn't know if he would be ready with the bag. It can be a long process to get back into that part of your relationship again. I didn't want to push it, but I wanted him to feel comfortable.

Sometimes recovery from that kind of surgery can take a year before you feel like yourself. My husband wears glasses and doesn't see well. When I said, "I am ready for it whenever you are," his reply didn't surprise me. "It's beige, you're beige, it's fine."

It felt different for about six months, even my pap smear was uncomfortable but now everything feels fine again—it just needed some time. I have a life now, thanks to my ostomy. We just got back into our routine and in our household; it's not a big deal. If we are going to be intimate, I make sure my bag is empty; it's a non-issue, and we've always been comfortable with each other.

—— ✿ ——

LUCKY IN LOVE
SUE (ANONYMOUS)

In the 1990s, routine screening for colorectal cancer was not practiced; any suspicions warranted a sigmoidoscopy, not a full colonoscopy. This was unfortunate for those with cancer further up in the colon. My doctor's mother died of colon cancer, so he was aware of the importance of screening and reminded me to get screened.

At the age of fifty-eight and married for twenty-one years, I received the news that I had cancer of the anus, news that only 1.8 percent of the population with malignancies of the digestive tract know about. The result was I had no choice but to receive a colostomy. The protocol thirteen years ago was radiation to shrink the tumor, then surgery with chemo before and after surgery. Despite the ill effects of these therapies, I am grateful for the daily opportunities I have to live life to the fullest and take for granted this good quality of life.

Back then, I thought I did things right with seeking two opinions. Neither of them told me that removing my rectum and anus would mean complications for the vagina, needing the support and cushion provided by the rectum. I wish the radiologist had told me radiation may affect the size of the opening and even shrink the vagina. Instead he told me only that he had "fried my ovaries." That didn't bother me, at fifty-eight years old I didn't need my ovaries, but I did need my vagina. Intercourse was painful, using a prescribed dilator was painful, and I could tell when using it that the pathway of the vagina was not straight, but slanted upward so any thrusting or pushing was not pleasant, and I felt sorry for my husband.

I am not very demonstrative when it comes to sex. I was raised as a Catholic in the '40s and '50s. In sexual matters I was never the initiator, but my husband was, in his quiet, gentle way. He thought at first that perhaps something could be done to change my vaginal problem. I sought help and sometimes he was frustrated thinking I had not done enough for myself. Sometimes I selfishly would say, "You don't understand!" We never really discussed how to have sex. When we both knew nothing more could be done, we simply accepted it.

I soon realized that I wasn't the only victim in this situation. I began to be more receptive to the idea that I could satisfy my husband through oral sex even though it is not something I would have chosen or relished. He appreciates it but sometimes apologizes; I assure him it is okay. We satisfy one another sexually. My husband is a realist and has shown such respect for me that I want to think of him and his sexual needs, and show him that same level of respect.

Because of my experience, I want others to know there can be unfortunate results with cancer of the anus. I needed to know more information from the surgeons, radiologists, and OB/GYN doctors about both short- and long-term effects of surgery, chemotherapy, and especially radiation. My questions were not answered sufficiently, and I did not understand the potential side effects associated with the proposed treatment for cancer. I would have liked to have been more prepared, but ultimately would not have changed my mind about having this life-saving surgery, even with the poor results that would affect our sex life.

Intimacy in our marriage has always included some hugging, kissing, fondling, and lots of endearing nick names. After thirty-two years of marriage, we aren't jumping into bed every week, but the thoughtful acts during the day and the reminders from my husband that I am the only one in his life makes life wonderful and worth living. He praises my courage and reminds me daily he loves me. I feel lucky in love.

———— ✒ ————

LOVE DOES CONQUER ALL
LISA WALDRON

After years of trying, my husband and I were elated to hear we were expecting. Our six-year-old boy would finally get a brother or a sister. Approaching five months, I didn't feel well. After a visit to the hospital, it was determined I had a urinary tract infection and was having contractions. Once admitted, I started on antibiotics and drugs to stop the contractions, but things only got worse. Even with the antibiotics, the infection progressed. On the third day, I lost my baby. I was able to hold him and get his handprints and footprints.

The doctors advised a colonoscopy to determine the severity of my situation. By the time they went in to explore, my entire bowel had seized and I was in kidney failure. I was twice my size due to fluid collecting in my system. It was determined I had toxic megacolon, a deadly result of c-diff (Clostridium Difficile). One of the doctors said I only had a 20 percent chance to live.

After waiting and fearing the worst, the doctors came out to update my husband. They were forced to totally resect my large intestine to save my life.

I was left with an ileostomy for at least six months, until everything healed. I have since had reversal surgery and am doing great. We are trying to conceive again.

My husband never ceased to amaze me with his overwhelming interest to help me feel better and be happy. He would eagerly look on as the ostomy nurse taught us how to change the appliance and care for it. He never hesitated to offer to help empty the bag and was better at changing the appliance than I was. He told me constantly he was happy I was here and he didn't even notice the bag. He still thought of me as beautiful and sexy.

I had a harder time accepting this lifestyle change, feeling like an alien with the small part of my intestine sticking out of my abdomen. I was filled with doubts, self-criticisms, and insecurities. He would say, "I still want you. I find you attractive, and you look perfect to me." He acted like it didn't bother him and he never wavered.

It's amazing how many people we connected with through this crisis in our lives. Our church made meals; they would offer to do housework, gave us blessings, fasted, and prayed for us. I think the prayers were healing. I had a doctor with excellent bedside manners who was caring and sensitive. When I was in the ICU (Intensive Care Unit), the pain was excruciating and I had a nurse who tenderly bathed me from head to toe each day; the care was amazing.

Fitness was important and I always felt connected to my body, but after ostomy surgery, I didn't want to connect. I went through cycles of depression; my husband encouraged me to go for walks. I was wearing sweat pants and baggy clothes. Ironically, I was probably drawing more attention to myself. Over time, we resumed our habits and my husband's main concern was to not put all his weight on me or try different positions to not hurt me. Even though I was turned off by the bag, he had no problem with it; he still wanted to caress me and touch me.

As time passed and I began to feel more secure, I realized I was given another chance, hopefully, left here on earth for a definite purpose. I didn't want to miss out on life and was happy we could resume a healthy sex life.

My husband once told me, "If I turned my back and let this event come between us, it would mean we were never in love. I love you with all my heart. Physical differences don't affect me; I see your beauty in so many ways." He would add wickedly, "I still want to do naughty things to you."

He makes me laugh, and I know he means it. I learned it was okay to be different and it could affect me as little or as much as I let it. The more time I gave myself pampering or dressing up really helped me rediscover my self-confidence and sexiness. I've learned I am all the things I was before and more—I am a survivor and a fighter.

This experience has unleashed my inner warrior. Knowing and remembering what I made it through keeps me grounded and reinforces that I can do whatever I set my mind on doing. Even with the long scar down the middle of my stomach, with the affection and continued support of my husband, I feel sexier than ever. Having had this painful experience, I am still richer for going through it even though it took a while to figure that out.

———— ☙ ————

EXCUSE ME!
Pam Bennett

I have had a colostomy since 1998 and have had some good, bad, laugh-able, and frustrating experiences over the years, but at the end of the day, it's enabled me to be where I am today.

We've been married forty-five years and able to maintain a sexual rela-tionship through it all. My close friend went to town and bought some sexy, teddie-type panties for me to cover the ostomy. She had the brainwave that if you put fasteners underneath, then all that needed to be done was unfastening them from underneath and you were away.

My husband, Ray, and I made a pact early on that if there were noises of flatulence, he would cock his leg up and say, "Excuse me!" He gets the looks and blame for any aroma. Our closest friends don't mind and once in a while will tease, "I think you need to simulate a fart, Ray."

———— ☙ ————

FEEL BEAUTIFUL
Cricket Henley

Seventeen years ago when I got my ostomy, I decided to buy a tube top from Kmart, thinking I would wear that when my husband and I were making love. The first time we made love after surgery, I wondered, *How am I going to feel beautiful and how am I going to be attractive to him?*

We took our vows seriously. He was so grateful I was healthy at that point. We began and it was good until the top of my bag came off the ring. My wafer was still on, but the bag was somewhere in our bed and my stoma was exposed. That put a damper on our intimate moment, a real buzz kill. I cleaned up, took a shower, and we started over. A week went by, we were in the mood and the same exact thing happened again. The first time I was worried he'd never want to make love again. The second time we just laughed about it.

I met my friend Lisa through a mutual acquaintance, and I was thirteen years ahead of her on the ostomy journey. She shared an idea she had about the Vixen Wrap. She wanted to feel better when she made love to her husband, so she designed a black ruched garment with pockets on the interior of both sides so the bag could stay close to the body without flopping around. If I would have had that on, even if my bag would have come off—it would have stayed in the pocket. It's like a crotchless cummerbund born out of a need.

We all need something that makes us feel confident and comfortable to be intimate. I had that tube top for fourteen years before I got the Vixen. Many of our customers from Ostomy Secrets wear it at night because it keeps the ostomy in one spot and not flopping around. We still want to have intimacy even if we have an ostomy.

Seventeen years ago, there was nothing. It feels good to be an advocate and be willing to be serious and silly. I modeled the Vixen at the first-ever UOAA lingerie fashion show. It surprised me when I just whipped off my shirt, me the daughter of a youth pastor, so everyone could see it and all I had on was a bra underneath. I am usually a very modest person; this was ground breaking and liberating.

--- ✿ ---

THE BAG MADE THINGS BETTER
Teresa Guzman

I am twenty-six years old and have been married for six years with the last four of those years contending with Crohn's disease. After a lot of rectal bleeding, fissures, and some complex treatment that only made things worse, I made the decision to have my colon and rectum removed.

I am extremely grateful to have my loving husband during these years. Before my health problems I would say that we had an average sex life, now life has been nothing but inconsistent, including our sex life. My husband is the one thing that has been consistent and stayed with me through the good times and the bad.

Once I had "downtown" pain, things came to a halt. Although we were unable to be intimate in a physical way, we became close in other ways. He would sit with me every evening when I got home from school while I took a sitz bath, and he'd sit with me again while I bathed before bed. Not being able to express our love in a physical way allowed us to open up in other ways. Also, there was no more room for privacy—he saw everything and it was definitely not sexy.

I read a lot of blogs and support group discussions online about people having troubles feeling sexy while they have a bag. People complain about it flopping around or being the elephant in the room. I have not had these problems. In fact, I think having the bag has actually made things much better. Maybe it's because I feel good again or maybe it's because I want to make up for lost time, but my bag has not stopped me.

I have ordered lingerie to hold it in place when I want to forget about it, but for the most part the only difference is that I might go empty my bag before we get started just so it's not an issue. Having an ostomy has made me more comfortable with my body, and now that I don't have any pain in my rectum or vagina, I am more appreciative that I can do what I want, when I want.

Having the bag has been good for me when meeting new people. I tell them right away, so I don't need to worry about giving an explanation when my stoma makes noise. This also helps weed out bad people who are disgusted or embarrassed. I think if I were dating it would be a good way to meet the genuine guys. If they can't handle a stoma and a little poo in a bag, then what else are they going to shy away from? My life is better because of having a bag.

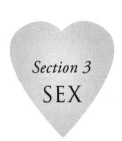

Section 3
SEX

Sex is emotion in motion.

—Mae West

The hypothalamus is one of the most important parts of the brain, involved in many kinds of motivation, among other functions. The hypothalamus controls the Four F's: fighting, fleeing, feeding, and mating.

—Marvin Dunnette

Sex is interesting, but it's not totally important. I mean it's not even as important (physically) as excretion. A man can go seventy years without a piece of ass, but he can die in a week without a bowel movement.

—Charles Bukowski

Sex is a big motivator for some people. Recently I found myself saying to someone, "I wouldn't doubt it if sex was in part some of the inspiration for the young Egyptians to overthrow their corrupted regime." They looked at me quizzically. I explained further, "In Egypt, the young men and women stay home with their parents until they get married. Many people can't get married and move on with their lives because they can't find employment. So they can't raise the necessary money to provide housing for themselves and their new spouse, so I am imagining that aided in the frustration of this awful regime." I don't expect CNN's Anderson Cooper will be calling me soon to explore this hypothesis.

We visited Egypt in 2011 and left just days ahead of the demonstrations to liberation at Tahrir Square. I had listened to my nephews who are in their mid-twenties in Egypt talk about their lives being on hold until they found jobs and could earn a wage to support a family. Many people in Egypt are college educated and still cannot find positions. My conclusion is that sexual frustration, combined with despair about the future and social media, offered a perfect combination for a revolt. Therefore, sex may have played a part in the revolution.

Years ago after I started writing a humorous medical column that came out quarterly, I started getting calls from people across the country who had read my articles. Often when they started talking I could tell they thought I had a medical degree and they might ask for help and expected I could answer their medical questions. I would tell them right away, "No, I am an ostomate, just like you, but if you want to go ahead and ask me, I'll see if I can steer you in the right direction." Often I would refer them to a consumer helpline at Hollister or look up the UOAA website and tell them about support meetings in their area.

One conversation still remains in my mind. It was a sweet, elderly gentleman with a southern drawl. "Brenda, my wife and I read your articles and we just love them."

"Well, thank you," I responded.

"I am wondering if you would be willing to talk with my wife. I don't think she feels pretty anymore since she got her ostomy."

"Why do you say that?" I asked him.

"Well, she doesn't seem too interested in sex anymore. I think since she got her ileostomy she doesn't feel attractive, and I can't convince her otherwise. It doesn't bother me at all. Would you be willing to speak with her?"

"Sure," I said, with some trepidation.

She came on the phone, "Hello, Brenda."

She sounded like a gentle, grandmother type. "Hi there, how are you doing today?"

"I'm okay, I love your articles—you are very funny."

"Well, thanks. Were you surprised your husband called me today?"

"Kind of …"

I continued, "How long have you had your ostomy?"

"Almost a year now."

She was so sweet, I tried to think about the best way to ask her the important questions. "How's it going? Everything working okay with your ileostomy?"

"Sure, no problems."

I took the plunge, "It seems like your husband is concerned for you. He's afraid since you had ostomy surgery that you don't feel pretty anymore, and you've lost your desire for intimacy because of it. Do you think that could be true?"

Indignantly, as her voice rose a little louder, "Is that what he told you?"

"Yes, isn't that it?"

"No, Brenda, he's totally clueless." Then with her southern charm she said sweetly, "Have you ever heard of the expression limp noodle? That's what I am dealing with here."

That took me by surprise but somehow I kept it together. "Oh, I see," was all I could get out before she continued.

"We even went to the doctor and got some Viagra and that other one and nothing happened."

"Oh, I see," I stammered again.

"I'll get him back on the phone again, Brenda; maybe you can talk some sense into him."

"Hello."

"Well, I had a lovely chat with your wife just now, and I don't think it's a problem with self-esteem and not feeling pretty in her case. She seems like she is handling the ostomy just fine. She says it might be a medical condition you have to deal with. May I suggest you both go see your internist or your general practitioner and talk this out? You do need a medical professional in my opinion."

"Okay, Brenda, we'll do that. Keep writing those funny stories."

"I will," I assured him.

Many of these stories divulge the will to keep on trying for this most primal instinct of sex. Some people have real medical challenges and yet that desire to have sex seems to filter through the challenges at times. For some people, it is a realization that their sex life as they knew it must change because of the surgery they had and the after effects. Sex seems often to be a benchmark to normalcy, even though at least one of the partners has an ostomy.

I endeavored to achieve representation throughout this book of a mixed population of gay, straight, married, single, older, and younger adults. After reading some of these inspiring stories, I thought to myself, *Maybe I better spice things up with my husband ... some nice rhythm and blues music, a scented candle and maybe we'll get lucky tonight ... if we can just stay awake!*

———— ⑆ ————

THE BEST RESPONSE
DAVE URI

Toward the end of my month-long stay at the hospital, I strolled the halls with my IV pole often, making my rounds saying hello to the staff and other patients, really just getting exercise. I would run into another patient who liked to stroll through the halls as well, and we would do a little dance with each other and our poles. We soon developed a friendship and exchanged phone numbers before being discharged.

We talked on the phone a lot over the next few weeks. I still wasn't feeling too well. I was learning how to deal with the ten-plus types of pills, and slowly getting back to solid food. While in the hospital, I got used to the TPN (Total Parenteral Nutrition) and medications delivered through my PICC (Peripherally Inserted Central Catheters) line (IV), and would have continued that had it been an option.

I had help making a schedule—it was tough figuring out all this while in pain and totally high on painkillers. My friend was rather immobile herself. She was in a wheelchair when we did our pole dances and was released when she could hobble on crutches. She had been in the hospital for something totally different from me—hurt both legs and an arm in an accident.

About two weeks later, we met at her home, just hung out, talked, and drank tea. We learned about each other's interests and talked about our past, present, and future plans. I could sense there was some attraction, mostly by a gut feeling (even though my guts were in a terrible state), and we both enjoyed each other's company and support during this hard time.

We continued talking on the phone and laughed a bunch. Being able to share the absurdity of our situations by laughing with each other was immense.

The next time I saw her, partly just for fun, and also because I figured it would be a good thing for our healing, I suggested we have sex. She considered it, agreed, and we each laid out our conditions (pun not originally intended). It was hard to make the first physical move, being careful not to hurt her, and feeling somewhat awkward, we got it going. I had never approached a romantic situation in this way before, and she didn't make it easy for me. I was in a generally weak condition, but she could only move one arm, so eventually we were kissing with me on top straddling her on the couch.

We decided to have sex before my surgery, and afterward. This gave us both something to look forward to.

I had no idea how sore I would be for the weeks following surgery. The second time having sex post-op, I suddenly noticed a different kind of slippery, and a smell. I was like, "Oh s--t!"—literally. My bag had slipped off and we were covered in s--t.

"*F--k,*" I thought, and she didn't even flinch. She just started laughing and I started laughing, too. We both cracked up and then headed to the shower to clean up. I couldn't have asked for a better response than that.

———— ✑ ————

A PROMISE IS A PROMISE
ALISTAIR OF SCOTLAND

I tell my story in hope that it can show you it's possible to get through whatever life throws at you, however hopeless things may seem. You can see the sun again and start your new journey to cope with the day-to-day trials and tribulations of families, relationships, and your new friend, the urostomy.

I was married for thirty years to the most wonderful lady. We have two lovely daughters, two grandsons, and as of this writing, two grandbabies on the way.

My wife and I and my daughter and son-in-law were out for a run one sunny day when my wife suddenly said, "I don't feel very well." She became violently sick and we made great speed to the nearest hospital. She was diagnosed with a brain hemorrhage and deteriorated over ten days until she was pronounced brain dead.

The preceding twenty-four hours before her death were more horrible than you can imagine. The only positive thing was that we were able to donate her organs, and she gave six patients waiting for transplants the chance of life. After her funeral, it took a long time for me to see any point in carrying on life; it was a real struggle for us all.

A short while later, my daughter announced wedding plans. Life continued, and I took on the role of Mum and Father the best I could. My oldest daughter then pronounced that she was expecting her first baby.

I had been attending my doctor with symptoms of a urine infection for some time. After the fourth visit, I pushed for further tests. This being arranged, I began to have severe kidney pain and was passing blood. Twenty-five years previously I had a tumor on my left testicle and had radio therapy at that time with no problems since. The doctor suspected I had a radio-therapy-induced tumor in my bladder that was blocking my ureter from my kidney. Because of the length of time I had suffered symptoms, it would most likely have spread. A CT scan and a biopsy was done to gauge the severity of the tumor, then followed an operation to remove as much of the cancer as possible. This was done via a hollow cystoscope through my penis. This would save my kidney and prepare me for chemo therapy and a later operation.

I was referred to the best surgeon specialist I could wish for and told that chemo therapy is not very effective against radio-therapy-induced tumors. They would double the recommended doses of treatment in the hope it would work. The cancer diagnosis was grave, and I had a 20 percent chance of living for five years.

During the long days of chemo, along with sickness and fatigue that accompanies it, my daughter was in great pain with her pregnancy, needing me to get up from bed to take her to the hospital. She lost the baby and it was a hard blow, but tempered by what was happening to me.

I came through the chemo, recovered enough by February, and told the consultant I was a fighter and intended to attend my daughter's wedding in May. He agreed to do the operation to remove my bladder, prostate, and surrounding lymph glands. He also promised to carry out a nerve-sparing procedure while removing my prostate to try and maintain my ability to gain erections.

Since my wife passed away, I had been emotionally supported by her closest friend. She introduced me to my wife all those years ago and was always part of our family. She has four girls and they are like sisters to my daughters. Some years before, she parted from her husband after discovering he had been living a double life. We had become close by now but found it hard to move on to a full relationship. It was difficult as we both felt we were betraying my wife. She was worried what people would think.

We went away for a weekend together the week before my operation. It was strange to sleep with another woman, but it was lovely to be together. With all the chemo and stress of everything, I just could not get an erection and that department was a bit of a failure. It was my last chance of things being normal before I embarked on my operation.

The surgery went well and I started recovery only to be knocked down by a serious bacteria found in my stomach drain, compounded later by blood clots in my lungs and a suspected heart attack.

My daughter was then rushed into the hospital very ill with the discovery she had an ectopic twin from the baby she lost earlier. She underwent surgery as they removed the damaged fallopian tube, and she recovered slowly.

My other daughter was at her wits' end traveling between two hospitals to visit us both. I spent six weeks in high dependency before I turned the corner and started my recovery.

There was a special nurse that helped me through. At one point I told her to turn off all the machines that were keeping me going; I had enough. The morphine had no effect on the pain, and it was giving me hallucinations. I saw my wife knocking on the window and shouting at me, "Fight! Fight!"

My final trauma was that after six weeks of not eating, my bowel had twisted. The pain was incredible and only relieved by a stomach drain.

I recovered quickly and kept my promise to my daughter for her wedding. I proudly walked her down the aisle and made my tearful speech after the meal. I danced the night away and collapsed into bed after. My lady friend went home with her daughters, as it was not openly known we were an item at that time.

After my operation, as feared, I had no erections. The nerve-sparing surgery had not worked. I was prescribed all the different drugs like Viagra and Cialis. Not even a tingle was felt.

For reasons mentioned earlier, my friend and I parted. She could not make a commitment and wanted to remain just friends. I joined a dating site on the Internet. I was on my own and needed company. I met a few people there and went out on dates, none of which worked out. I then met a lovely lady and we spent nine months seeing each other most days. She understood about my stoma and inability to have full sex.

My surgeon suggested I try injections to see if they would work to give me an erection. It was a bit embarrassing learning to inject my penis with three nurses looking on. It did raise my manhood a little and, with an increased dose, it did work to a certain extent. We tried it out for a while, but the nerve pain was so severe, it was not pleasurable. You say to yourself, *I am lucky to be alive and sex is not that important.* I still think the same as you can have plenty of fun with a willing and understanding partner.

Months passed and my wife's friend started to get back in contact with me. She said she had changed and missed me terribly and wanted me back. I was fond of the other lady but could not see a future with her. I tried to let my newer partner down gently and went back to the lady I had known for over thirty-five years. That was hard; I felt a real cad.

Life carried on with surgery to repair an incisional hernia. My surgeon suggested I have an inflatable implant placed in my penis. I researched this on the Internet but could not decide if that was a wise thing to do. He referred me to a specialist who described the procedure at great length.

My lady friend thought I was mad, but I made the date for the operation. It was a two-day stay in the hospital described to my daughters as "a fix down below." They did not ask too many questions and left things to me. It was all fine but so painful, and I wished I had given this one a miss. After the swelling receded and I was told to inflate the apparatus, it seemed to be the very solution. That was two years ago and although I can have intercourse, it is not anything like the real thing.

It is a big decision to go for this procedure, as any normal function you may have is lost forever. The male feeling of arousal is lost although you still climax, or rather have the feeling of climax. It always feels cold now, as the blood flow is reduced. You can use a vacuum pump and fit a restriction ring with care, but it is such a procedure that it takes away the moment. Intimacy is all about closeness and feeling wanted by a partner rather than ego. I am a very tactile being and need touch.

It's been four years since treatment and the cancer has not returned, thank goodness. I spend every weekend with my new lady and we are very happy. One day we will sell two houses and get together for real. It's hard to make two families into one. My surgeon refers some of his patients to me if they want to ask any questions about their stoma operation or the sex side of things. I am a member of the stoma association and have volunteered to talk things over with anyone that needs advice and help.

During my journey, I found a great pen friend in the USA who has had a stoma operation as well as MS. She is an angel and gives me so much inspiration to carry on. I would have floundered if not for her help and support with relationships and just life. I have found that by being open about having a stoma people will ask if I will talk to their friends and acquaintances for advice or just a supporting chat. I do that when I can and many an idea to help has come from simple discussions. I trust my story will help others as well.

—— ✿ ——

PUP TENT SURPRISE
BOB BAKER

The surgeon went over the options with my wife and me prior to the procedure to remove the colon cancer. I was in shock as most newly diagnosed people are—this was a big decision with too much information. One of the risks I remember hearing about was the possibility of impotence if I had my rectum removed. *No thank you*, I thought. *I think I'll keep my rectum.*

I was admitted to the large, teaching hospital and given good care. The surgery went well, lab results were good, all that was left to do was heal up and go home. I am a light sleeper and had trouble getting any real solid rest, probably due to the fact that I lived with ulcerative colitis for so many years. For most of the stay I was awake when they arrived every two hours to check my vitals. They had given me an epidural for the surgery, which was in my back, for three days to relieve the pain, along with a Foley catheter to handle my urine output. When the time came to remove the Foley, they sent the youngest, most attractive nurse they could find. Naturally, I was embarrassed, but glad to be free of the catheter.

It was the fourth night that I finally gave in to sleep—no more tubes or lines. They brought me a sheepskin mattress cover and I was feeling comfy. I must have been dreaming of some soirée in front of a fire wrapped in sheepskin when all of a sudden the lights clicked on and two young student nurses stood at the foot of my bed staring at me. They both had a hesitant look on their faces and as I followed their gaze, I realized what was going on. I had pitched a pup tent.

We got through the embarrassment, they took my vitals, and left. I may have been their first "camper" that night but probably not their last. To be honest, I was just happy it still worked.

—— ☙ ——

MY COVERALLS
CINDY SYLVIA

Looking at myself in the mirror of the bathroom, three days after surgery, I remember staring aghast at my image and thinking to myself, *who would ever want to love me, really make love to me?* I knew my parents loved me, and I had friends who cared for me, but I don't mean love in that sense of the word. I wanted love in the sense of mad, wild, and crazy romantic love that makes your heart skip a beat and fills your head with obscene thoughts that make you blush to acknowledge.

As a young lady of twenty-five years, I had been dealing with ulcerative colitis for six years after having bathroom issues since I was a child.

In my career path, I had been student teaching when I was forced to withdraw from college to take time off again to cope with my illness resulting in ostomy surgery. In previous summers I had been a nursing assistant, and after having been in the hospital as a patient, it was obvious that elementary education was not for me. My new plan was to attend nursing school and get my degree, then on to a training program to become a WOC Nurse. Two years later I graduated, went to work at the very hospital where my surgery had been done, and after getting a couple of years of work experience with the esteemed surgeon who did my ileostomy, I left to go to a hospital in DC, fell in love with the area, and never went back to Boston.

As the years went by I became a confident young woman, experienced in the ways of life, and living an independent life in a brand new city. My surgery was simply a fact of life, part of whom I was and who I was becoming.

I was engaged a couple of times after surgery and the stoma was never an obstacle for my love interests. The next man that came along was a winner and a keeper. Although younger than me, we were mutually attracted and he says he knew right away. Before long, we were together all the time. I knew we were getting more intimate in our relationship, and I wanted to make sure he knew about the ostomy. I told him, "Before we get too close, there's something you need to know. I was sick for a number of years, and I had a surgery where they rerouted my bowel and removed my anus."

He said, "Oh, you have an ostomy? I dated someone before that had one. It's no big deal for me. Is it for you?"

I had built this up in my mind that this was going to be a problem, but it never became one. For whatever reason, I never faced a rejection because of having an ostomy. I consider myself lucky. My ileostomy never seemed to faze him and at age forty-two, I got married. When it came to sexual intimacy, he was happy with sex at least once a day, and I am in the groove now, too; my ostomy has never been an issue.

I have always been meticulous about my appearance, my wardrobe, and my ostomy pouch, though not visible to the world, was now a permanent part of my anatomy, and I wanted it to be as attractive as the rest of my body. After all, I owed it to myself to maintain my image, not just for others, but for me. It made sense, just as I wear a scarf, a pretty pair of earrings, or a sexy bra, that I had to have a special piece of lingerie to wear over my pouch.

Since I am not a seamstress, I found a lady who could create unique artistry with a needle and thread. I started marketing my pretty pouch covers and named them My Coveralls. I would change my covers to suit my mood or outfit, and I thought other people might enjoy that, too. I always wear one; the only time I take it off is when I take a bubble bath. I feel absolutely naked without it.

It's the pouch that needs the lingerie. Let's face it, when the pants come off, and especially while making love, I want to feel sexy. Each cover is unique, some with feathers, and ribbons made out of rich, quality material with a variety of colors. My favorite is a whimsical, gauzy, black pouch with black and silvery fringe and tassels all over it that flows in the breeze, if given that freedom. They contribute to making me feel confident and wantonly attractive. As long as I feel that good, nothing can stop me. That's why I wanted to share them with others like me who have ostomies. We need to feel the best we can about ourselves and a pouch cover can add to the mood of the evening.

It's been thirty years since that day I looked in the mirror, and I never looked back, but at the same time, I will never forget my experience as a patient. By the way, my heart still skips a beat when my man walks in the room.

———— ✄ ————

FROM LUST TO LOVE
FRED SHULAK

As a gay man living with an ostomy, there were times I talked about it right out front and other times I chose not to. There were only two occasions where I have had unpleasant experiences. The first time I was in my twenties. I met a man in a movie theater. We were both attracted to each other and wanted to spend time with one another. We had known each other for only minutes and there was no mention of my ileostomy. At that time in my life, I didn't make it a point of mentioning it beforehand. (That changed over the years.) We were just two horny men who wanted to be together. When we got to his apartment, it didn't take us long to get into bed. Before long, his hands ended up where my rectum had once been. By this time he had seen my appliance so I told him, "What you are looking for, I no longer have available." He apologized and said that he was looking for one thing and one thing only—anal sex. He apologized and we parted company.

The second incident was when I met someone online about sixteen years ago. He was from southern Wisconsin, and he was coming to my house to spend the evening and morning. When we started making love, I suddenly realized I had a small leak in my pouch. I excused myself and explained that I had a problem, and it would take a few minutes to fix it. He didn't seem deterred by it and didn't ask any questions. The evening wasn't ruined because of what happened, but we both knew we were not that interested in each other and didn't bother to maintain further contact.

I met my partner in 1996, at a function hosted by a local Bears organization. Bears are not like the Lions or the Elks clubs. A bear in gay society is a man who is happy and comfortable being very overweight. He prefers to be bearded and not clean shaven. A bear prefers denim pants, flannel shirts, and overalls. Bears are very often into leather, sadist and masochistic relationships, as well as slave and master scenarios. Bears are known to be kinky and are closely allied to leather.

Sean and I were without a doubt the oldest guys there. I was fifty-eight and he was sixty-one. His wife had passed away from cancer two years prior, and he was exploring the alternative side of his nature—something he had denied himself his entire life. We exchanged telephone numbers and e-mail addresses.

When I got home, I immediately got on the computer and was going to send him an e-mail. I thought to myself, *Boy are you a jerk! Here you just met this terrific guy and didn't do anything about it. Are you looking for the white knight on the white horse? This is an opportunity that you shouldn't pass up.* I got my courage up and called him and we made arrangements to have dinner the following night at a restaurant near his house.

Our dinner conversation was a generic getting-to-know-you conversation. However, he mentioned his wife had been rather sick with ulcerative colitis and had an ileostomy. A couple of years later, she had problems again and required additional surgeries and each time they took out more of her small intestine. Finally she was diagnosed with Crohn's disease.

I commented that the ileostomy is a good option to get rid of the UC, but that Crohn's is an insidious disease that will never be gone—at best, might go into remission. He looked at me quizzically and asked, "How do you know so much about ileostomies, colitis, and Crohn's?"

The time was right and I told him, "I was diagnosed with UC at four-years-old and that for the past forty years, I, too, have had an ileostomy."

After that night, we started seeing each other on a regular basis. It was my busy season, and I had to work on Saturdays. Consequently, I would spend Friday night with him, go to the office on Saturday, and after freshening up at home, would go back to his place on Saturday night and stay until Sunday night. Sometimes he would come out to the suburbs and spend the weekend at my house or come to see me in the middle of the week and go to work from my place the next morning. He had a small dog to concern himself about and on the occasion when he spent time at my house, he would bring her with him and then drop her off at his house before going to work.

Because the ileostomy was no stranger to him, we had a comfort zone that could not be surpassed. We dated for seven months before we started living together. One night I said to him, "You were happily married for thirty-five years before your wife died. We have been seeing each other on a regular basis for several months now. Do you consider yourself to be heterosexual, bisexual, or gay?"

Without hesitation he emphatically said, "I'm gay."

I asked him, "Do you still like women or are you afraid of women?'

He replied, "I like women and I'm not afraid of them, but when it comes to sex, I'm gay."

We had a close and nurturing relationship. We were together for fourteen years until he passed away from cancer in 2010. I miss him every day.

---- ⊛ ----

TOMORROW IS ANOTHER DATE
JON O'NEILL

Up until July 2010, our sex life was pretty good with lovemaking two or three times a week consisting of two warm and fluffy morning-in-bed sessions and maybe a last-thing-at-night along with the occasional outdoor kerfuffle to liven things up. I might even go all out with bath, candles, incense, and a bottle of cava (Spanish champagne), followed by a slow body massage. The outdoor stuff is either on mattresses beside the pool or a knee trembler in the pool.

At the end of June 2010, I had major surgery for stage III bowel cancer and ended up with a permanent stoma. The wound in my bottom took eight weeks to heal and then a final six sessions of chemotherapy began. Chemo makes the bag completely unpredictable. The treatment is four hours intravenous followed by fourteen days of tablets with a week off before everything starts over again. In the last few days of the week off, I begin to feel better.

It has taken time to not be embarrassed by the bag. My wife says she hardly notices it. I did try a plug during what I thought was a quiet time. I got ready, plug in, white boxer shorts on, lying on the bed, when all hell broke loose. There was a rumble from below and the plug shot out like a popgun in a cartoon. The end of what was to be a romantic time. I am going to try irrigation after the poisons have left the body.

Aside from the bag, if that is not enough, the chemo has done something to the main attraction. What was a happy relationship between mind and nether regions has now become a diplomatic lockout. In good times, I could raise an erection at a drop of a hat or a saucy thought. Now, erections are like gold dust and hard to find. I can think all the raunchy thoughts I like but nothing happens. Even when we are active, I don't know what is going on below. Nearly all feeling has gone. The only way to get a rise is to have manual manipulation by my wife. Even after penetration and minutes into what should be a happy conclusion, I get a message, there will be no explosion and it is frustrating. If an ejaculation occurs, it is more of a letdown than a fission of joy.

My last idea was to change the timing altogether. I proposed late morning. No bath (bag embarrassment), no cava (alcohol may have a diminishing effect), a minimum size cap in place of a normal bag, just the massage followed by sex. The first time, it worked a treat. Tomorrow is another date. Wish me luck.

———— ⊗ ————

FIXED PAIN BECOMES MIXED BLESSING
Maria Barker

I had my bladder removed two years ago after having lived with bladder incontinence my entire life. When I was younger, my father took me to several doctors who informed him I was a lazy child and should be punished every time I had an accident. After that, each time I had an accident, I was smacked.

I shared a bedroom with my older sister and had two younger siblings who, thankfully for me, were babies. Most nights their bedding was soaked too, and my mum showed me and my sister how to change the bedding and include it with the other wet sheets from the babies. I was also sent to school every day with a little bag for my soiled underwear and another for my clean knickers.

That's how I managed it most of my life. It wasn't great and only got worse as I grew up and began to date. My incontinence had gotten worse over the years, and I attributed it to the stigma I endured as a child. Truth be told, I was terrified I would be found out. I became good at hiding it by wearing babies' nappies, which I would cut down to fit me, and I would always make sure I had spare underwear with me. I still had accidents, but I could usually fob it off with different excuses like, "I waited too long in the loo queue!"

In April 1983, I met my husband. I thought he was my knight in shining armor. We'd been going out together for a few weeks when I told him of my embarrassing problems. "I have no control over my bladder," I admitted.

I went on to explain, "I don't know why, but I had a lot of problems with my kidneys as a child and chalked it up to the fact that I can't control my bladder." I was scared to admit this to him because I had lost a lot of boyfriends because of this problem.

He was different, and I felt I had to be honest with him. I was twenty-two years old when we married. He was in the army and we'd been posted to another country when my husband asked me, "Why don't you speak to a doctor about this?" I told him, "No way!" I had never gotten over the ridicule from the time I was a young child.

A year later I was rushed into the hospital with a massive kidney infection. I expected I'd be given a drip antibiotic and sent home. This time it was different. Besides an infection, I had scans done the following day, requested by a urologist who informed me, "We need to get to the bottom of this to see why you keep getting such severe infections."

Within forty-eight hours I had surgery to remove my left kidney. I thought we were nearing the end of it when the doctor pulled the curtain aside and asked me, "Maria, how long have you been incontinent?" I was shocked. I tried to deny it, but my husband spoke up. "She's been like this her entire life."

The doctor explained, "Your bladder is very deformed and scarred. I might be able to help you." Then he sent in a nurse who taught me to catheterize myself, but it didn't help.

Soon I fell pregnant and, boy, did I have problems. Now my incontinence was not only involving my bladder, but my bowel, too. When our son was born, it was a relief, but short lived. Because I was leaking urine constantly, it was decided I would have a hysterectomy. I practically begged the doctor to take out the bladder; I had been dealing with pain for so many years.

I plodded along. My husband finally came out of the army over four years ago and by then I was fitted with a supra-pubic catheter, which was good, but extremely painful every four weeks when it had to be changed. It was very sore.

Three years ago my urologist admitted me to the hospital to try to do something about my bladder. When I woke up from surgery, my God, did I know he did something different. When I signed the consent form, I was informed that if my bladder was rotten and couldn't be fixed it would have to be removed because it was a constant source of infection for my only kidney. When I awoke my surgeon explained quietly, "Your bladder has no muscles, you will never have control over it and it was so badly scarred, I had no choice but to remove it." As devastated as I was, I have to say that for the first time in my life it was great not to be sore down below. Finally, some relief.

The next day my husband was visiting with our son when the nurse asked if she could check the wound. When I looked at my husband's face, he was horrified. Even though we'd been given a leaflet about having the bladder removed, he said to the nurse, "How long has she got to have that?"

The nurse said, "For life."

My love life changed that day. I saw that look on his face, and I had a sixth sense this had seriously affected him. I was discharged from the hospital two weeks later and, for the first time in my life, I had control over my urine. That was amazing for me but bad for him.

The first time my husband and I went to make love, it was horrible. He kept telling me, "Turn the bloody light off, I can't look at that thing!" No matter what we tried with different positions, we could hear the bag slapping against my stomach. I tried to wear a t-shirt over it to see if that helped. I found that either lying on my side or by having sex with me on all fours, he still hated it and kept telling me, "Can't you take that thing off?"

We had been together a total of twenty-seven years. I trusted this man, I put up with him calling me names and acting like a pratt. I supported him when he had post-traumatic stress syndrome, when he treated me like dirt, then two weeks before Christmas in '08, he announced, "I don't want to live with you any longer, and I've been e-mailing my girlfriend for over a year."

I was gutted. I couldn't believe this kind, gentle man who had never once been nasty towards me before surgery turned into someone I no longer knew. Just before he left, I asked him, "Why?"

He said, "I hate that bloody thing on your gut, and I want to have sex with someone who's normal."

I felt alone when he left; I was scared to let another man in my life. At first I hated the bag, but I credited it with saving my life. The surgeon told me I would have died due to the chronic infections. I'm forty-seven years old. I live in the United Kingdom. I'm not very good looking, and once in a while I would think, *who would want a woman with a bag attached to them?*

Recently I was told I have to see a nephrologist, as it seems the infections affected my renal function. This comes as no surprise to me; after all, you can't be incontinent all your life without it affecting some organ.

My soon-to-be-ex has a new girlfriend and decided to tell her all about his wife who, as he put it bluntly, "Does nothing but piss herself all day long." My ex can sod off for all I care; I'm happy now. When I married him, it was for better or worse. I put up with him ridiculing me and making me feel like my stoma was something that should be hidden. He actually did me a favor by leaving. There are a lot of ignorant people out there, but it gave me an inner strength and now I have a life that doesn't involve sitting in a pub almost every night. I have a new life, and if I am lucky enough to meet a good man, then one thing is certain, I have a stoma that gave me a life I'd never known for over thirty-six years—it saved my life and I am proud of it.

My grandchildren came to visit, saw my pouch, and asked, "What are these?"

With my future daughter-in-law's permission, I explained to this lovely, little five-year-old that I can't pee like her and then I showed her my urostomy pouch. Keira asked several questions, and I answered the best I could. Now she tells her friends, "My nanny Ria has a special bag, and it helps her because she can't wee wee like me."

Thanks to my granddaughter, I was asked to go into her school to see the head teacher, as Keira was very upset when a little boy called me names. With the parents present, I was asked to give a talk to the children. At first I was scared and didn't know what to say, then with a little help from my son, I told the children about my special wee wee pouch. I took along several items that I use to change my pouch. Questions followed from the children as well as the parents about my urostomy pouch, including questions about my childhood. I answered them honestly.

After the talk, all the children crowded round my granddaughter and now she has lots of new friends. Just as I was packing up, a young mother came to me and asked if she could speak to me privately. We went to one side and I asked, "Is there something wrong?"

She told me, "I am twenty-six years old, and I can't control my bladder."

I felt so sorry for this poor girl. I asked, "Have you done the pelvic floor exercises?"

She nodded yes.

"How long has it been going on?"

"Three years," she said quietly.

I gave her my urologist's number. "Go see your general practitioner and if he isn't any help, I'll see what I can do."

Later I found out her doctor basically fobbed her off. Thankfully, she told her husband, who was very good. Recently she had surgery and now has complete control of her bladder. I am so happy for her; I just wish someone had helped me when I was a child.

As for me, I haven't met any men, and I am getting used to being alone. I hope my story can help someone else who may be like me who lived with this dirty little secret, which wasn't really a dirty secret at all, but a condition that was not my fault. Thankfully, the medical profession has come a long way and if my story helps one person, then I've achieved something good out of this. I just started going out to bingo, who knows—I might meet a man over a bingo board!

———— ⊗ ————

LEARN TO BE FLEXIBLE
Patrick Tobin

I had some challenges with erectile dysfunction for the first year after surgery and also had some challenges with the acceptance of the bag. I had ulcerative colitis for twenty years. The last five went downhill rapidly.

My doc said, "Your colon's coming out in six months. You decide when."

Surgery was four years ago, and I tried many bags before I finally got the Hollister products to avoid leakage between appliance changes.

The first challenge was getting it up. I had an ileostomy, but the surgeon left the anus and an inch and a half of the colon. I could not get an erection. I talked to my regular GI (Gastrointestinal) doc, and he prescribed a round of Viagra and also said this was not uncommon due to all the poking around the surgeon had to do. Well the pill worked; however, the morning-after headache felt like a hangover headache. But it was worth it. The need for the Viagra has, for the most part, passed. It's still fun, and if you take the pill early enough in the evening, the headache is not nearly so bad the next morning.

The other big challenge was getting my wife past the bag. Those see-through plastic drainable jobs will kill any intimacy. Between the view and the noise, it was not good. We have finally worked through to a comfort level where I can either use the small closed bags for in-the-buff action or the underwear with the removable crotch panel if I just put a new bag on and don't want to throw out the new bag. It can work if you are flexible and willing to try new things.

—— ✥ ——

YOU CAN SURVIVE A LOT

Sari Mogol Legge

July 16, 1987—The doctor stopped in the night before surgery that was scheduled at 6:00 a.m., "You ready? Need anything?"

"How 'bout a bottle of tequila?" I asked.

"No, but I can give you a medical buzz," he grinned.

"Then get me so high that I can bend over and kiss my own a-- good-bye!" I weighed eighty-seven pounds, and he prescribed enough to knock out an elephant, yet I was too hyper to sleep. At 5:00 a.m., I got up and showered with my old body for the last time.

My dad had died on Father's Day, one month earlier, from prostate cancer. Everyone in the family was a wreck. I spun the surgery to relatives, assuring them it was going to be great, trying to make *them* feel better. I was only twenty-six years old, a rock radio announcer, and all I wanted was to live life with '80s Cyndi Lauper-colored hair and all.

The surgery removed the rectal passage, my entire colon, and a bit of small intestine, too. After years of being deathly ill and in and out of the hospital, I had hope for my body to recover, even though I knew it would be an arduous effort including physical therapy for six months.

On August 9, my mother died at the age of sixty-three, following my dad by just two months. By October, all my hair fell out from the stress, malnutrition, and body healing while coping with the deep loss of both parents in one summer.

My body healed. It was the first time I had been healthy in a decade. My spirit also healed by attending a twelve-step program. I learned I needed to work on a lifetime of co-dependent issues. I came to understand that my marriage was abusive, irreparable, and possibly deadly.

In 1989, I ended a seven-year marriage and began to explore my readjusting self-paradigms. I wanted to recapture lost time, have a second childhood, and be the rock-and-roll princess I imagined for myself. With a mental flip of a switch, in ecstasy of being alive, I had an attitude of *Damn the torpedoes— I want to live life fully!*

My ostomy allowed me to be sexual, being freed from illness and isolation. I was calculating as I selected someone deserving of my sexual favors. I liked being in control. Now I got to party and enjoy being the hard rockin' radio chick. Not great personal choices, but it was a helluva lot of fun. I could drink anybody under the table. I could squeeze forty hours into a twenty-four-hour day. I was unstoppable—a legend in my own mind.

My ex-husband repeated often, "No other men will want you after you have this operation." I set out to say f--k you to him and the disease. I would explain to a male conquest, "My body is an exotic rebuilt chassis that saved my life and allows me to be with you. All the parts that you want are ready and able."

As they questioned me, I gave them an education explaining it as an upper, not a bummer, that it was an attraction, not detraction. At which point I'd take their hand over the pouch area outside my clothing and I'd say, "Do you feel that?"

"Yeah."

"That's the change. I have no colon, my illness almost killed me, and this is the cool science that makes life and love possible."

"What is it?"

"It's my waste management plant … I'll show you if we are going on from here."

Whatever the mojo I had—a nice young body, confidence, my sexual aggression—only one man made the wrong comment and was rejected by me.

I eventually calmed down and enjoyed three serious relationships, each raising my own standards. I became selective and learned I had to love and respect myself first rather than seek external approvals. Even though I learned a lot, my heart was broken a few years later, and I fell back into filling the void with alcohol and having sex without the emotional attachments.

I never thought my body would allow a pregnancy to carry a child after years of illness and body changes. A friend with benefits conceived my son with me through two forms of birth control and on the second time we had sex. A month later, no period missed, I fainted in a business meeting. A girlfriend got me a pregnancy test, and as the plus sign appeared on the stick, a grin spread across my face. The entire lake heard me through my open bathroom window—*Whoo-Hoo!*

The OB/GYN had concerns and no experience with an ostomy pregnancy. All my prenatal tests came back healthy. God was blowing angel dust on this pregnancy. This was a miracle. The earliest ultrasound clearly showed a boy. I began using his name, Jacob Israel. From the moment I was pregnant, it was all about my son. I missed sex, but I was in love with being a mother and doing it right. The birth was rough, but I had a healthy son, my gift, Jacob.

I joined a dating service when Jake was nearly four. I wanted to go to a movie and a dinner with someone whose food I didn't have to cut, and some much needed adult conversation. My judgment had been bad in the past and the service chose dating candidates for me. It was a new business, and they screened everyone with a criminal background check and found compatibility. With a child to protect, I was approaching life differently. Hooking up in bars was no place to find Mr. Right.

I am 5'2" tall, and the dating service picked a 6'3" ginger-haired Englishman.

I didn't go out with the Englishman for a long time; we had glorious phone conversations, hours long, and I loved his Yorkshire dialect. He met all my standards—didn't live with his mother, owned a business, right age, and no children. He was too nice, *what's the matter with him?* I found out the good guys do exist. At the same time, I didn't realize the Crohn's was back doing internal destruction.

When I finally agreed to go on a date, I immediately fell for him, but I was thinking, *I'm just horny.* Peter knew immediately I was the one for him too. I had told him right away that I had Crohn's disease, but for the first time, I was worried about how he'd feel when I told him about the ostomy; I was afraid to tell him. I had decided I was just going to be a good friend; I didn't want to lose him. I put off sex and we had great make-out sessions, which led to revealing my ileostomy. He didn't care. I still hesitated; years of saying yes too fast did not work out for me. Yet, he kept showing up, bringing pizza, and playing with Jake.

My health was in distress again, surgery was necessary, and I was scared for Jake. I couldn't predict this cycle of illness or how it would compare to my younger years. On top of that stress, I was about to lose my job, too.

My family took care of Jake while I had an emergency stoma revision done in Minneapolis. Peter would close his shop, drive 3 hours daily from Nisswa to the Twin Cities to watch me in a drug-induced sleep even though I was unaware he was present. He was a keeper, and also the first man my family and friends ever liked and encouraged us to be a couple.

With everything happening, we still had not been sexually intimate. After surgical healing and the two of us getting emotionally close, I knew it was time. I brought him back to my home while Jacob was in day care. I grinned widely as he took me after four years of no action. Prior to Peter, orgasms didn't come easily, but Peter rung my bell that night and it's been ringing ever since. He became Jake's dad, and we married in England in 1998. Peter remains the love of my life and father to Jake.

Over the last fourteen years, it hasn't always been easy with my health and making a living. I was finally granted full SSDI (Social Security Disability Insurance). In 2008, we nearly broke apart with cumulative damage of hardships and have since recognized mid-life crisis contributed to that awful time.

With menopause, I felt like I had no sense of self. Fighting depression, I made a good show of walking and talking, but Peter and I withdrew from each other and almost lost it all. I didn't feel like a woman and no longer cared about sex or anything else. Peter wanted sex, but I had no desire. We went through hell and have come back together through therapy and use it as a necessary tool. Self-learning continues, both of our esteems were battered, our lives separately and together had to be reexamined and given respect.

I cannot lie. It is not the ostomy; it is auto-immune complications that we must deal with even when it is hard on everyone. As I enter into my fifth decade of life, my ability to be a woman and cherish who I am has nothing to do with my ileostomy. It has to do with continual work to love myself so I can live and love to the fullest for the time I am here in this life.

------ ⊙ ------

LOVE'S STRENGTH TRIUMPHS
STEVE GOLDBERG

In November of '95, I got engaged to Heather and the next month I started having stomach pains. We were both getting our masters degrees, and I was living away from home when my life started collapsing in front of me. I wasn't able to hold on to a conversation or get to places on time. I knew where all the bathrooms were, and I was unable to drive long distances.

For a few months there were misdiagnoses at the hospitals. I quickly lost a lot of weight. My mornings started at 4:00 a.m. for a 9:00 a.m. class. Waking up in pain, I didn't always make it to the bathroom in time, and then I would wait for the bloody, painful stools to be over. My fiancée, Heather, witnessed my screams of agony and would try to comfort me knowing in five hours I had to be sitting in campus. It was a stressful start to each day with trying to eat a pop-tart or cereal, drive myself to campus, find a parking spot, and run into the building to find a bathroom again before class.

One memory of a trip to Blockbuster lingers. I told the clerk, "I have to get into the bathroom right now."

"I am sorry sir; you have to go up front to get the key."

I had no control, and I crapped my pants right before I got into the bathroom. Everything I was wearing was ruined, I had to leave the store soiled, and Heather drove me home. I had to sit in the back seat facing backwards, the pain was so bad.

I was on my death bed and we had not been married yet. I was still trying to get my masters in school counseling, and I found out one of my professor's daughters suffered from Crohn's disease about the time I was finally diagnosed.

"Steve, you are going to die if you don't get your colon out," said the doctor. "The ulcerative colitis has eaten through your entire colon. It has got to be removed or you will die."

My surgery took place in December of '96; I only had to lose two months of school and was fortunate to have professors who understood my situation and were compassionate.

I am so thankful Heather stayed with me. When you suffer through something so painful and questionable and you don't know what's happening to your body, you need someone that loves you while you are at your most vulnerable state.

We hadn't been intimate for what seemed like forever, but is now a mere blip in time. It's almost impossible with ulcerative colitis; when the body is moving, waking up in the morning, just after you eat, your body triggers the pain/colitis. When it came down to wanting to be intimate and have sex, it had an initial detrimental effect on our intimacy.

After the surgery, I was cut from the belly button and through my rectum with my rear end sewed up. My privates were a purple-brown-bluish color, and I was scared I would not be able to have sex again. Heather was present when I came to, and I was able to speak to her.

"My God, you better ask the doctor what is going on. With things being a different color, am I going to be able to have sex again?"

They laughed it off, assuring us the color would disappear and that we'd be having sex in no time.

Heather was helpful in so many ways. She would make sure I had the proper dressings and that my spirits were up. She didn't do hands-on care. She's comfortable talking, standing by me, hearing me scream, and holding my hand. I needed to learn how to take care of myself. When it came to the emotional and intimate side, there was an unspoken change. The person she agreed to marry was free of health complications; now I have a pouch of poop on me at all times.

She suffered emotionally as a caregiver. She was a strong woman even at twenty-four; she had gone through difficulties in her life and knew emotional pain. One way it affected her was the worry over not knowing if her husband was going to die and also thinking of our future children, knowing that there was a chance they could end up with ulcerative colitis.

My WOC Nurse was amazing—bringing both of us in for a visit, she made a big difference. She had an ostomy herself and connected me with the UOAA and the youth rally and urged me to come in to be a counselor for this association. "With your school counseling and your life experience as an ostomate, you can absolutely help." She talked to us about having sex and having children and played an important role in my recovery.

I was anxious to have sex again. I remember the doctor said, "You are cured; it's a matter of recovering from surgery now. Don't worry, it will return to normal even though we had to cut a lot out."

In our first experience, there was no discussion, just a matter of having an erection. There were logistics to work out, the clip from my ostomy pouch jabbing her, or while having sex, when I hit the wrong angle, or moved too fast, having that clip dig into my testicle could kill our lovemaking. Depending on the position we're in, my pouch can make noises every once in a while. We just laugh it off.

We were a passionate couple and became closer, our bonds stronger. Appreciating being alive, intimacy isn't all about the sex. With more than a year passing since we were able to cuddle for any length of time, sex came later. Having the surgery opened my eyes to reach out and touch the lives of many other youth and adults that have suffered. It feels great to know I could make a difference.

This is who I am now—I wouldn't trade it for anything. My two young girls know their daddy has a pouch. There is nothing I can't do because of this pouch; I continue to be active, and take on anything that interests me emotionally and physically.

If you wrap your mind around the end results of the surgery, you're golden. If you wrap the pouch around your mind, you will be in a hole and never get out of it—plus it would smell bad!

——— ⊛ ———

ORDINARY IS GOOD
Dawn Becker

I was dating someone for a while, and we were getting closer. One day I was wearing a cut-off shirt that showed my abdomen and revealed a scar.

"How did you get that?" he asked.

I explained to him that I was sick for a lot of years with ulcerative colitis. He had never heard of it, so I told him my story. At age twenty, I was in and out of the hospital for three years dealing with ulcerative colitis. The nurses thought I was a junkie because I would lose twelve pounds in two days and they'd ask me, "What drugs did you do tonight? How much cocaine have you taken?"

It was so frustrating that they would never believe me when I came in dehydrated and very ill. In 1988, when that was going on, there wasn't much known about the disease. I was in and out of the hospital for three years. My gastroenterologist was trying everything to help me avoid surgery. Things would be under control for a while and then I'd get another horrendous flare-up. Stress seemed to make the problem worse.

After I told my boyfriend about my history, he wanted to know why it happened. "No one in my family has a history of this," I told him. "The only thing the medical people could tell me is that it was a nervous disease."

My boyfriend was much more disturbed to hear about how rudely I was treated by the nurses than worrying about me having a pouch. Becoming intimate was a little awkward. I was worried. I wanted the lights off. I wore a tube top around me so nothing would show.

"Why do the lights have to be off?" he would ask. "What's the big deal? It saved your life; I don't care if you have a bag." He was not bothered by my ostomy, but I wasn't comfortable with him seeing it.

Later, I married a pharmacist and we've been married eleven years. I have a whole drawer full of tube tops, and I still prefer to not show my bag. In the first conversation I had with my husband about my ostomy, I explained it more clinically and as a matter of fact than I would to others because he had medical knowledge. When I could tell we were getting closer I said, "I want you to know that I have an ileostomy because I had ulcerative colitis."

Knowing what an ostomy was, he was very interested and fired off a few questions. "What meds were you on? What was your treatment plan? Why didn't a reversal work for you?"

"My colitis was too far gone and there were not enough healthy intestines to save it. In 1992, I walked into my surgeon's office and told him I am having the surgery with or without you. It's too much. I'm not getting better; in fact, it's getting worse, and I want some quality of life. I begged my doctor for an ileostomy."

I considered myself lucky. For my husband, it was okay—no big deal. Our love life is very ordinary. Once in a while when we are being intimate, my pouch will make a noise and he'll make a noise right back at it, and he has totally accepted it. We own two pharmacies, so he even orders my pouches for me. We have been blessed with four children and all of them were natural deliveries. I am grateful the man I married is a pharmacist who cares for me and understands my medical condition.

———— ☙ ————

LUCKY IN SEX
BIG TREV (ANONYMOUS)

I was on holiday ten years ago on the Mediterranean island of Malta with my wife, mother-in-law, and brother-in-law when I began to feel severe pains in my stomach. With language difficulties, the local chemist prescribed something to help control diarrhea instead of something to take care of constipation, and my problems became worse. Within two days, the pain returned with a vengeance and was so severe I was almost driven to distraction even with taking painkillers by the handful. We left the next day to return home, and on the way, I was told I ranted and raved and remembered nothing of the flight, the wheelchair, or even being loaded into the plane via a forklift. I acted as if I was drunk and didn't remember any of it until two weeks later.

My in-laws had persuaded the family doctor to come to the house, and when he arrived, he made the quick decision to get me to the hospital without even waiting for an ambulance. Within one hour I was in surgery, and it was determined I had a perforated bowel due to diverticulitis.

When I awoke in intensive care, I found out I had been on life support for two weeks, and now had a permanent tracheotomy and a colostomy. My wife hardly left my bedside for a moment while I was in the hospital. The wound I was left with was so huge it took almost four years to completely heal. To top it off, I lost forty-five pounds and was also told I was a diabetic.

Prior to all this, my wife and I enjoyed a full and varied sex life. It was a few months before I was able or even felt like making love. Now that I felt distinctly physically unattractive, it took courage to make the first move. When I eventually did, my wife said, "Don't ever make love to me if that bag is full."

This was disconcerting because my self-esteem was quite low. My wife was never good at coping with medical matters. I never blamed her—there are lots of people like that, and it's not her fault. We did continue to have a sex life of sorts, but inevitably it led to friction and, unfortunately, due to this and other problems, we separated over four years ago. I must accept the blame as, in retrospect, I probably expected too much.

All my life I have been a part-time musician playing guitar and keyboards in bands and recently in a one-man band. About six months after my colostomy operation, I started performing but couldn't handle the vocals as well anymore because of breathing difficulties, and I was no longer getting the pleasure out of it as I once did. I still work as a boiler man part-time and have had no problems with my stoma for over ten years. It's all the after effects that I've had trouble with and can't seem to win.

Nearly three years ago, I met Anne and we started dating. She is the most understanding person, has a lovely nature, and is extremely kind. Anne is very attractive and twelve years my junior. She has no problems at all with my imperfections—physical or otherwise. She doesn't mind changing the dressing on my wound if necessary and even wanted to know how to change the colostomy bag if the need would arise someday. I am now having the best sex of my life—you name it and we do it. I can't believe how lucky I am that things turned around.

Section 4

CAREGIVING

You give but little when you give of your possessions. It is when you give of yourself that you truly give.

—Khalil Gibran

Things turn out best for those who make the best of the way things turn out.

—Jack Buck

When I was diagnosed with colorectal cancer at age thirty-nine, I was a caregiver for my two children ages three and five. I also cared for my staff and my clients at my busy hair salon, and when I had left over energy, I even cared for my husband. I was an independent career woman, mother, and wife whose world changed the moment I found out I had cancer. I soon learned what it was like to be the care receiver.

Finding out I had cancer of the rectum, I learned life-saving surgery would require a hysterectomy, permanent colostomy, and vaginal reconstruction. I, who had never once thought about my bowels or their very function in life, suddenly was thrust into a world where ulcerative colitis, Crohn's disease, and cancer would now become part of my regular vocabulary. I would learn over time that many people with bowel diseases had endured horrible pain for years. I felt like I was one of the fortunate ones—I only had cancer.

After being diagnosed with cancer, I was immediately surrounded by people caring for me in new ways. My friend Sherry was the first to arrive with a home-cooked meal and a listening ear. When she found out I would be required to have an ostomy to live, she internally freaked out. Her own mother had an ostomy after being diagnosed with cancer and all she remembered about it were the accidents and awful smells that emitted from that time.

Sherry accompanied me to a couple of appointments and watched me shed a bucket of tears in five minutes of pity party time after each invasive test. I could count on Sherry, my mother, and a few other girlfriends to come along with me at each scary test or scan. My husband usually stayed home to care for our children or else he was at work. English was not Bahgat's native language and medical terminology can be difficult and I wanted another set of ears to hear what the doctors had to say to me. I welcomed the women in my life along to listen in and ask questions for me as my mind often wondered to any place but there.

My own experience of caregiving took on many different aspects as a patient. My husband provided stability by going to work each day and making sure the kids were at the day care and picked up when needed. He was very attentive at the hospital when learning about the surgery I would be going through. Never once did I feel he was rejecting me for having an ostomy, the early menopause I would go through, or the months of recuperation with the reconstruction that I would need. He was compassionate and ready to pitch in with wound changes or pouch changes and always with a positive can-do attitude.

Family helped out often and filled in when others could not. Dad and Mom were my sounding boards and the people I let see my tears. My girlfriends helped take care of my children. Many different friends took turns coming over at 7:30 in the morning, hours after my husband had left for work, pulled me out of bed, then made breakfast for the kids, got them dressed and my son off to kindergarten. In the meantime, I would take a shower, change my ostomy pouch, get dressed, and after two hours of working up a sweat, I would end up on a chair where I would stay for the next few hours. My job was to heal, and it was all I could do most days.

Our caregiving team extended to my neighbors who watched my children after school and my Bible study group from church who provided meals for the family. My husband still talks about those delicious meals. And there were friends that vacuumed, did my errands, and played with the kids. We had a village of people caring for us.

I noticed the various ways people reached out to help us even though I was in a cloud of pain medication and self-obsession that revolved around getting the pouch to stay on my deteriorating skin and the poop from flying out everywhere. I had a flush stoma and stuff was going under the pouch instead of into it. At first it was a constant battle as the doctors and nurses tried to help me solve my ostomy issues. They cared for me the best they could. That first year was tough, adjusting to the ostomy, and then it was followed by two stoma revisions within a couple of years—more life threatening surgery that yielded the same kind of stomas. I wondered if I would live until age fifty at one point. I had self-esteem issues and worried that I would never heal or be able to have a normal life again. Slowly, over time, my body healed and my soul followed. Prayers and learning how to irrigate my ostomy helped too.

Not everyone is blessed with friends or extended family that can help out in times of need. Some people are afraid to ask for help and don't let anyone know how they are suffering daily. We often think we have to be totally independent and take care of ourselves and we can take a long time to heal physically and emotionally. People love to be asked for help, especially the people that care for us; they just need to know what to do.

In the following stories, there are many examples of caregiving and even a couple that don't involve partners. One story talks about how a daughter provided just the right care and another credits her animals for motivating her to heal. Friends, partners, and even a grandson round out the richness of these tender stories and as the quote by Jack Buck says, we make the best out of the way things turn out. Most caregiving anecdotes in this book have to deal with primary relationships and the daily needs required when dealing with an ostomy, but there also comes the necessary time to care for ourselves, to feel as secure with our ostomy lifestyle as we can.

The more caregivers I talked to over this time preparing this book, the more I realized that their roles are often exhausting, relentless, and underappreciated no matter how much they are loved or how much compassion they have for their loved ones. We, as patients, especially in the beginning of our times with our new ostomies, require a lot of attention as we learn to cope with the mechanics of an ostomy and the daily rituals.

It is important the caregiver gets a break too, or perhaps they will burn out way too soon and not be able to take care of their partners or themselves. It's like the old metaphor of the oxygen mask on the airplane when the flight attendant says, *do not assist others until you have placed the mask on yourself.* How can our caregivers continue to give if they are not nourishing themselves?

A while back, I had a friend in her forties who died of ovarian cancer. She was divorced and had young children and relied heavily on two friends that were married with children of their own to provide most of her care toward the end of her life. My job was to take care of the caregivers by providing some comic relief, a place to vent, and an occasional glass of wine or a bit of chocolate. It wasn't much, but it helped care for them when they were giving so much of themselves to her.

This last year was a tough year for both of my parents who needed care. Luckily I have seven siblings who live nearby, and we were able to take turns caring for them. My father became septic and almost died, and he was the major caregiver for my mom who had dementia for fifteen years. He had to have months of rehabilitation and wasn't home for almost a year. Not everyone could spend the night with Mom, but some could spend a couple of hours, prepare a meal, grocery shop, or wash clothes. There were many laughs shared with Mom and she often accompanied us on our various errands, which always included visiting Dad, along with attending children's activities. She was almost always pleasant company and loved visiting Dad, always thinking she hadn't seen him for a long time when it was usually just the day before.

Sadly, we lost Mom to a massive stroke in January 2011, but no one has regrets for not getting to spend time with her. My father recently commented, "As tough as it was being in the nursing home recuperating and away from your mom for all those months, I kind of got used to being by myself for hours at a time, and now I am a little more prepared to be alone. You kids each got to spend time with Mom, and I know she enjoyed that very much, too. And we were together for a while before she had the stroke. It's amazing how things turn out sometimes."

He often sang to her and she'd sing along, "On Top of Old Smoky"… or "I'm in Love with You, You, You," and each night they had a ritual where they would say their prayers together. Eventually Dad had to say Mom's part too, and at the end, Dad would tell her, "I love you, and everybody loves you."

Dad is adjusting to her being gone, but he says it's the little things he misses. He reaches over to cut her ham for her in the morning and then realizes she's gone on to a better place. My father still teaches me as he shares those precious moments of living with losing his wife of fifty-six years. Caregiving becomes a gift of grace at reflective moments like that.

Nationally, as ostomates, we have the United Ostomy Association of America whose purpose is to educate and advocate for people with ostomies, to help them see the life-enhancing and life-saving surgery as a new beginning. They extend their national hand to the individual chapters who in turn are created to serve the needs of the individuals with ostomies. Sometimes as people with ostomies, our greatest service is to reach out to another person with an ostomy, to give them hope and lead by example to living life with joy.

—— ⊛ ——

INSTANT ATTRACTION AND LASTING LOVE
CARLA AND ANTHONY ANDERSON

I met my husband, Anthony, at the funeral of a mutual friend. After the gathering at the house with food and socializing, Anthony was seated at the table I was cleaning. He said, "A woman after my own heart."

I was just helping a friend, doing the woman thing. I was instantly attracted to him, and I pursued more information about him to find out where he lived. I wanted to know if he had a girlfriend, so I started hanging out with people in his apartment complex. At that time I was going through a lot and I was really looking for affection. He was hot, cute, and attractive, and I started learning more about him.

He had a job, didn't have a girlfriend, had his own place, and I moved in on him and knocked on his door one day.

He's not a talker, not very social, more of an observer. He can sit in a crowd of people and likes to observe, so I initiated talking to him.

Before I met Anthony, he was an automotive fabricator, the hose man. He enjoyed it and did a lot of work under the hood on the movie *Too Fast, Too Furious* and has been recognized on the TV show *Monster Garage* along with being well known for fabrications for Harley Davidson and DUB accessories. He has done community service for the local fire departments and park and rec vehicles, and has been able to custom make those hard lines for those restoration projects. He has made quite a name for himself that has traveled across the United States.

We first started dating seven years ago. After I tracked him down, we used to get together and go out to the bar, play some darts, and drink a little bit. When we started making out, it only went so far and seemed to be more of a one-sided thing. I was more the receiver; he was pleasuring me and wouldn't let me give in return. I knew something was up, but I didn't know what. We hung out in the same crowd of people and no one ever mentioned there was anything different about him. He was a little reserved for a while, and I wondered why he wasn't pushing for sex.

Prior to meeting me, the discouragement and scare of trying to initiate a relationship or conversation was difficult because he was always concerned about what was going to come down the road—concerned that no one could love him with a bag.

We were at his place in his room and I finally asked, "What's wrong with me that you don't want to go further?"

At first it was hard for him to tell me, "I had cancer."

Being the inquisitive type, I wanted to know all the details. At last he opened up and explained the type of cancer he'd had and all that he went through with the colon cancer. It was a ten-pound tumor inside his colon and the surgery left him with a colostomy. He received chemo and radiation together, which burned his bladder away, so they built him an Indiana pouch, an internal bladder that requires him to catherize.

Doctors flew in from everywhere to witness this surgery. He was one of the first to have a colostomy and Indiana pouch at his age. They recorded it, videotaped it, and it made many medical books. His biggest fear about the cancer was losing his hair. The breakdown from the radiation deteriorated his small bowel, and the result is painful never-ending fistulas. Out of twenty feet of small bowel, he only has three feet left.

I found it didn't bother me at all. Maybe that's one of the reason he loves me so much—because I showed him it didn't bother me. There have been times when it's frustrating, where the bag has broken and we just go to take a shower. It bothered him a little bit, but the more I reinforced it was going to be okay, the easier it got.

When he told me about the cancer, I was already so infatuated with him and liked him so much. My next comment was, "Let's go to the toy shop."

He was unable to have an erection. At one time he was using an ejection but that was over ten years prior.

He was able to work many years and then four years ago, they had to take the small bowel after an obstruction, and then he got sick and has been unable to go back to work. Since then he acquired another fistula in the crack of the butt, and he now has a bag that hangs from his crack.

He's lost his job, his social life, darts, and can't sit down, can't even reach the bag to empty it himself. He's lost so many things. I fight to keep him out of depression. He feels like he is keeping me down because I want to take care of him. We are drowning financially, barely above water. It's hard and the most difficult thing I've ever gone through because he's my best friend. I see the stress overwhelming him as he has to stay in bed and watch life go by.

I felt like he had the right to have a family and a wife, and I was the one to be that for him. What keeps me here is my willingness to care for him, make him comfortable because I love him. He touches so many people's lives socially, from work and medical people who break down and cry because they see what he's going through. The sympathy is overwhelming. He has been such a productive member of society. He didn't crawl into a hole, and he keeps fighting to live.

We can't even hug while we are in bed because he's in a lot of pain; just a little pressure hurts him. When he sits and stands, it hurts him, but he's a warrior; he keeps going. I can't get us in a stable place to live. Even my children from a previous marriage are living with my mother and father while I care for him. We have not been able to financially keep it together where we can get a place for all of us to stay together, and he wants that. His illness has robbed him of being able to be a dad to his ready-made family.

Mom and Dad have seen the change he's brought into my life. If it weren't for him, I'd be in a different situation and probably self-destructive. He always lives on the edge of death and it's humbled me. A lot of bad things left me because I was able to be with someone who cared about me. He looks at the world differently than I do because of living so close to death. In a way, I am saving his life and he is saving mine. We make an impact on people around us because they perceive our relationship as the one they want, as an enviable relationship.

He gives me strength. I've been beat down and gone through a lot and been very alone. I was a waitress and started going to school to be a nurse, which is my destiny. Now I know I wish to be an ostomy nurse someday. My husband's given me a sense of security. I am capable, rather than being told that I'm a loser. He tells me how beautiful I am. I couldn't have been blessed with a better man, and I'm thankful for him and his love.

—— ⊛ ——

CAREGIVING GOES TWO WAYS
ANDREW BAKER

My wife lost loads of weight and blood as she dealt with ulcerative colitis. Our sons were two and four, and the doctors told us that my wife would not make it without a blood transfusion. We are Jehovah's Witnesses. We don't use blood, yet we wanted the best treatment possible. My wife got on a saline drip and steroids, and I was allowed to bring in toys for the lads so we could stay with her.

The stoma nurse was a man, and he was brilliant in telling us about the ostomy. He showed us a film and gave all of us, including the lads, a sample bag to stick on, which we did. Once again it was explained to us that Vanessa could die if she did not have this life-saving operation.

The doctor was concerned about doing the operation without using blood, as he had never done it. He kept his promise and did the operation without transfusions and afterward we went to thank him. Instead, he thanked Vanessa because he learned he could do the operation without the need for transfusions. He told us he did the same operation to another lady on the same day and he used blood and noted that she was in the hospital two weeks longer than my wife and did not heal as quickly.

Life was different after the operation. Vanessa was no longer tied to the bathroom; she put on weight and looked healthy.

We were young starting out together. I was sixteen and she was fifteen when we got married. There was family stress and in those early days I was horrid to my wife. We were not Witnesses yet, and I wanted a divorce, but somehow we got past it.

Vanessa comes across as a hard person, although she is very caring but hides her feelings and never cries. She always says, "What does not kill you makes you stronger." I wondered if the trouble I caused her made her stronger. She has been a great wife and mother. These days I am in a wheelchair. She has a good career but finds it hard that we are caught in a system where if she works we lose money. We never know how much help I need in the day as some days the pain is too much, and yet, she copes with that.

Since her operation, her sleep suffers since she always slept on her tummy. She is marvellous in the way she deals with her ostomy and carries on like it's not there. The only challenge is the smell, and she hates going away or using someone else's toilet. In our house we have two, so she can have one to herself.

Over the twenty years with her ileostomy, she has had a positive outlook since there is no more pain. When we were younger, a lady made Vanessa a band of material to hide the bag; it was not very effective, but it gave us a laugh.

About fourteen years ago we came to Ireland where the company decided to do away with the product my wife has used all those years. Trying to get different supplies here is not so easy, but my wife takes it in stride even though she has sensitive skin.

With life, there has been good times and bad ones, but the one thing we managed to do well is bring up our two lovely lads that everyone seems to like. I hope I have changed over the years, and every day I am grateful Vanessa stayed with me.

———— ✇ ————

LET OTHERS HELP
CAROL LARSON

One of the most difficult challenges to face in a long-term illness is to let your children or close family member take over the role of being your caretaker, if even for a short time. It doesn't feel natural when it's usually been the other way around. But there may be times in your life when you don't have a choice.

I remember an incident years ago, when I started my chemotherapy treatments. After a somewhat invasive diagnostic procedure, my husband drove me back from the doctor's appointment, and left for work after I told him I was okay. After he left the house, however, I experienced trauma, both physically and emotionally from the procedure.

My daughter Tami called me on the phone and noticed I was slurring my words. I know my brain and body felt like mush.

She offered to come over and I replied, "Absolutely not. I'm just fine."

Nevertheless, she was at my door in fifteen minutes.

According to her, I looked like the kiss of death. She immediately made me drink some apple juice, and when we sat down in the living room, she noticed my hands were cold and had a bluish tint to them. I started to shiver, so she grabbed a comforter and put her arms around me. Tami wanted to call an ambulance, fearing I was close to being in shock but afraid to leave. Instead, she rubbed my hands and instinctively started to rock me like a baby, humming to me. The extra warmth and the juice did the trick. Within twenty minutes I was better. I had stabilized and the crisis was over.

I often wonder what would've happened if Tami hadn't come over when she did.

Looking back on it now, there have been other circumstances when I just had to let go and let others come to my rescue. I can honestly say it took a whole village to sustain me: my family, my friends, my neighbors, my doctors and nurses, therapy, and my support groups.

People have said to me, "How did you get through this ordeal so well?" And I reply, "I had help—lots of it."

———— ⟨⟨⟩⟩ ————

NO ONE DOES IT LIKE SKIP
CHERIE DeGROOT

You know that movie *Alien* when the creature came out of the stomach? That was what I looked like after my stomach blew up and was septic, leaving me with a wound big enough for my husband, Skip, to put his whole fist into it. I died twice on the operating table but for some reason, I came through.

Two months before this happened to me, Skip was paralyzed from the neck down for four days. He recovered, but only 80 percent. He never had a chance to concentrate on himself to get back to normal before taking on the role of being my caregiver.

For eighteen months I had to be hooked up to TPN (Total Parenteral Nutrition). The process took fourteen hours daily and required me to push my IV pole to the bathroom several times a night. I lost eighty-five pounds, going from a size fourteen down to a size two with no strength or body fat left and was exhausted.

Skip hooked up the TPN and helped me change my ostomy bags because they were at an angle I couldn't reach. He has been my rock; I don't know what I would have done without him. Skip quit his job to stay home to take care of me, organized my prescriptions, and even made the meals. We needed to do this for months while the recent J-pouch built inside me healed.

Skip was by my side through my nursing home and hospital stays, and each time he learned a little more about my care, like cutting my pouches so they would fit properly and last longer. I had many complex problems, saw many specialists, and on one particular trip home, my bag started leaking. We were at the end of our rope and both of us were totally exhausted and felt defeated. The insurance didn't pick up my supplies and they were costing us over $1,000 a month. It would be a while before Medicare would kick in.

"How can we keep this up?" I asked my husband. In exasperation, I said, "I want to go home and kill myself. I can't handle this anymore."

He looked at me and in all seriousness said, "We'll do it together." Skip was worn out too.

"You would?"

"I can't imagine living without you. Let's just give it some more time and see if things get better," he said resignedly.

I think a guardian angel was on my shoulder because we didn't go through with it even though we discussed it. We had lost contact with friends and family; our lives revolved around this illness for three years. We couldn't afford to have a home health agency come in and do this for me every day. We had been married forty-four years when I was allowed to be on social security disability after being terminated from my job at the hospital. Skip was a retired fireman and had a job delivering flowers, but had to stop that to take care of me. He couldn't go hunting or to basketball games because he had to be with me. I finally qualified for Medicare, some of the pressure was off, and we were able to get some more coverage for expenses.

Once a week I would have lab work done and my PICC (Peripherally Inserted Central Catheters) dressing changed. There was a doctor there who had reviewed my case. No one wanted to touch it because it was so complicated. At one point we had two bags on my abdomen dealing with fistulas. We'd go through ten to twelve bags a day. My husband would sleep on a chair or couch. For months, we didn't sleep. The doctor told us that I was one of the most difficult cases he'd ever seen.

There have been times when my husband wanted to leave with all the stress financially and emotionally. One time we got into a big fight, and he said, "I can't take this anymore," and he walked out. He felt guilty and came back. Skip had to put his life on hold for a while. We get along much better now; the fights were a build up, blow up, then over. Sometimes at night, he'd be watching the news and say, "I don't want to hook you up right now, I just want to watch TV." I didn't blame him; I hoped this bad time would soon become a distant memory.

Intimate relations have been at a standstill. I don't feel sexy yet. Sometimes Skip might say, "I need a hug" and that is the extent of it. I write in a diary and all my frustration comes out there. It's the only place I allow pity parties.

Things have been slowly getting better. Months later, the fistulas finally healed along with the J-pouch. We both have a sense of freedom again. I realize now I had taken so many things for granted—a simple walk, a swim in the pool. This summer I'll be able to get my bathing suit on again. Having lunch with a friend or Skip going to a game—it's the little things we love doing. We hold our breath still, afraid it's too good to be true.

It will take a while to get over that trauma, but we are looking forward to putting it behind us. My PICC line just came out two weeks ago and it was great to be able to take a shower without plastic wrap protecting everything. We had to laugh when Skip said, "I actually miss doing the IV feeding. It was a real routine for us. I miss the time with you and going through the process." I think it made him feel he was worth a lot to me, and he still is. We definitely communicated more as a couple because of it.

On the first day without the PICC line, I suggested we have the breakfast of champions. "Let's celebrate with having Bailey's Irish cream and coffee." We enjoy the independence again and we learned a lot together—especially to never take things for granted. And I learned what a blessing Skip is to me. Maybe that was the reason for everything.

———— ✥ ————

I AM BLESSED
CHRISTINA SOWALL

When other little girls brought their purses, they likely contained a little plastic mirror, hairbrush, and a fake tube of lipstick. I would never leave the house without mine full of toilet paper. I had signs of IBD (Inflammatory Bowel Disease) since I was at least two years old with constant tummy upsets. Diagnosed with Crohn's, ulcerative colitis, and erosive gastritis when I was twenty-two years old, I got treated with medication and moved forward.

When I got married in 1978, my husband knew I was sick and took me anyway. In 1986, I had my first bowel resection and lost one-third of my small intestine.

Then, while living abroad in the UK and Malaysia for ten years, I had another bowel resection. They kept me awake, and I observed them dropping the IV on the floor and they started to put it in my arm. I purchased another one with cash on the spot.

We moved back to the USA, and I was sick for quite a while. There was a surprise fiftieth birthday party planned for me, but on the way to the restaurant, my husband took me to the ER instead after I passed out in the car. The supposed two-hour surgery turned into eight, and I woke up with a colostomy, ileostomy, and urostomy—three bags.

The urostomy was reversed shortly after, but I elected to keep the other two because for the first time in my life I felt free. I wasn't running to the bathroom eighty times a day.

My husband, Keith, was the kind of man who, although we had three children, would never change a dirty diaper. He drove the baby to the babysitter to change the diaper.

And then I came home with ostomies. This red-necked, six-foot tall, brawny, electrical engineer, red-headed, bearded, masculine, hunter-fisherman, who rebuilds cars and is a man's man, really impressed me, especially when he is standing in front of me and I shoot him with poop. He'd take it all over, wipe me down, and start all over again. I was shocked, totally shocked, and never expected that from him. He accompanied me to every appointment, and, for over a month, that man changed my ostomy appliances, often getting squirted along the way. He never flinched and he never disappointed me. The first time I changed it myself, he was a little saddened that I didn't need him anymore.

He continues to support me. I never throw up the red flag soon enough, I always feel I can handle it. I won't let the disease get the best of me, so I go too far the other way, and he has learned to recognize that about me.

He bought an RV so I could see America with a traveling bathroom and that is the ultimate support. Watching my every move, he'll ask, "Are you okay to go out to dinner? Are you okay to take this hike?" He provides me the opportunity to back off.

After surgery, I asked the surgeon, in front of Keith, when we could be sexually active again. The answer was, "As soon as you are comfortable with it." She set the guidelines of avoiding certain positions to not hurt me.

Within a couple of days we were establishing a new routine. We went with the positions I used when I was extremely pregnant, and they worked really well for us.

I had gone on the Internet, preparing for when I could be intimate. I purchased crotchless ostomy panties that came in two pieces that held the bags and came with a pair of panties for every day. I would go to bed with that ensemble, and. if the opportunity presented itself, I whipped out of the underwear and then I was left with the crotchless panties with the section that held the bags. The colostomy was more like a giant band aid pouch that didn't need any attention.

That's gone now, too, because they took my colon a few years ago. My surgeon is a woman, and at my bedside after surgery, she let us know that she left four to six inches of stump in my rectum and then she just winked. We hadn't asked about it before, so she just let us know that in case we wanted to use it, she had left it for us.

Having the ostomies was never much of an adjustment. I had preplanned the special panties and that helped a lot. When I get my night clothes on, I change my underwear into these special panties. We are always spontaneous, so I wear them every night, and it is a great benefit to both of us.

This experience with ostomies opened my eyes to how supportive and close Keith has been and that caught me by surprise and I am blessed to have him. I am five-foot-six inches, fair, blonde, and a straight forward person. I tend to have a positive outlook and forget negative things. We have three kids, blessings from God. I was told I couldn't have children or carry a baby to full term because of IBD. After the third one was born, the doctor advised me to stop having children.

I have been blessed with supportive siblings and children too. I am currently the president and executive director of the IBD Quilt Project that creates awareness of IBD and all things related. I was an art major and have a stained glass studio and do it now on commission for family and friends. The connections I have made with people because of having ostomies have been very meaningful and changed the course of my life. As I said, I am blessed.

———— ✍ ————

LIFE IS IMPORTANT—LIVE IT!
DAWN VANDER HAAR

I put off getting an ostomy as long as possible. After fifteen years of dealing with Crohn's and three surgeries, I feared I wouldn't be a normal woman anymore. I was afraid I would not be able to wear nice clothes, that I might stink, or have my husband of twenty-nine years not want me anymore. I was sick for many years and with so many pre-cancerous polyps showing up with my scopes, I was given no other option. I talked a lot to my husband about this and how our life would change, but he and my two daughters said they wanted me well and around for a long time. After surgery to remove my colon, it was discovered they got all the cancer so I didn't have to do follow-up treatment.

I refused to show my body to anyone for months and went into a depressing time for the loss of what I used to be. I had felt totally unsexy for two months and then one day my husband grabbed my hand and took me off to bed and made me feel like the woman I used to be again. I always try to cover the bag with a teddy during sex and make sure my bag is emptied; sometimes I don't eat ahead of time when the sex is planned. Once I get over the embarrassment I'm okay, but sometimes I try to at least cover the bag with my hand. He says it doesn't bother him and tells me it's about me, not the bag.

I am still leery of what to wear and change the bag every three days just in case others can smell it. Sometimes, I just want my skin to breath so I take an hour-long bath.

Do I wish I didn't have it? Yes.

Am I glad I'm around to see my kids and grandkids? Yes.

Thankful I was in a loving, caring, marriage before this happened? Yes.

Would I remarry or date if something happened to my husband? No.

Life is worth living. It's not what they take from us; it's what we do with what is left that matters.

    —— ☙ ——

FAMILY ACCEPTANCE
DOUG MILGRAM

My seventeen-year-old grandson took up fly fishing this year, so we drove to the mountains to find some trout. We ate breakfast at the lodge and planned to fish a hole about a mile away. Like most teenagers, he inhaled his food. I'm a slow eater, and as I finished buttering my toast, he asked, "Can I go fish the hole behind the lodge until you are done with breakfast?"

"Yes, I'll come down when I'm finished," and off he went. Shortly after, I grabbed my rod and I set off to find him.

There were others fishing the same hole, and I found him on the other side of the river. Since I don't wade, I told him, "I'll fish here until you feel like coming around."

About that time I could hear those funny noises my stomach makes, and I felt a slight pull on my belly. Figuring I had plenty of time to get back to the lodge, I waited for him. Just as he started back, there came those sounds again, only this time I could tell they were wet sounds. My belly got heavy, and I thought, *Self, you better haul butt to the nearest john.* Climbing over the river bank, I felt a gusher. When I stood, everything ran down my leg and started coming out of my shoe as I walked, leaving a tell-tale trail.

I am smart enough to leave an extra set of clothes and pouches in the car in case of trouble; my problem was I drove the truck. Right before we left, my grandson asked if we could fish a hole that was up a road, which required four-wheel drive. Forgetting to transfer the emergency bag to the other vehicle, I was now soaked, I stunk, and the stuff just kept coming.

I thought about wading in the stream, but at this point the river comes out of a seventeen-mile-long limestone cavern, and the water stays at about fifty-three degrees. I did accidentally step in the water and the light tan stuff started floating down behind me. If I had gone in up to my waist it might have been fish kill, possibly gotten a citation for polluting the stream.

God bless my grandson Christopher who knows about my ostomies, what they are, and how they work. For a while he walked behind me and kicked dirt or stones onto whatever dropped from my pants. He distracted people that were standing around so that I could get back to the truck without notice. A few looked at me a little funny. I think they could smell something strange in the air. Luckily, I had rubber bands in my vehicle and I secured them on my pants around each ankle. I really can't say I don't know what I would have done without my grandson because without him I wouldn't have been in the mountains in the first place!

Once in the truck, I was safe, but the grandson wasn't—he had to put up with the smell for the two-and-one-half-hour ride home. He even asked to stop at a Mickey D's and was very polite as he said, "I think I'll go in and eat, and would you mind not eating until we get home?"

After arriving home, I got out of the truck, took off my shoes and the rubber bands, and walked into the shower fully clothed. I forgot about my cell phone and it got wet. My first wife, Elaine, (I like to tease Elaine, referring to her as my first wife, even though she's the only wife I've ever had; I get a little kick out of watching the reactions from others when I introduce her as my first wife) told me that if my phone ever got wet, I should stick it in uncooked rice, so I did. At first it would automatically dial sixes or bring up the Internet showing an error message. After sitting in the rice and sunlight for a few days, it worked fine.

When we were sitting in the doctor's office before the urostomy surgery, the doctor asked how our sex life was since this surgery was probably going to hurt it.

An old joke came to mind, and I put on a big grin, stood up like I was happy as all get out and said, "We have sex once a year."

He fell right into it, looked at me kind of funny, and said, "If you only have sex once a year, why are you so happy?"

I said, "Tonight's the night!"

During my urostomy surgery the doctor went snip, snip, and snipped the end of my sex life. I swear first wife paid him. Now instead of chasing her around the house for a little lovin', I'm content to read the newspaper. I met Elaine in June, and we were married two months later. After forty-five years of marriage, it's taken me this long to get to know her.

My wife has shown her love for me every day in many ways over the years. Six years ago I was around the marina a lot and the owner suggested since I was always hanging out there I might as well work for him. I jumped at the chance until he said it would involve staying there some nights when he was out of town.

At that time my urostomy was new, and I was having a tough time changing it myself so Elaine always helped me. Since I didn't want to be eighty miles away and spring a leak, I asked her if she would mind staying up there those nights with me. This was only a few times a season and usually on the weekend, but one time it was in the middle of the week. Without a blink she left work, drove the eighty-five miles, got up at 4:00 a.m., and drove the eighty-five miles back to work the next day.

For many that might be a standout, but for me, it's just Elaine. That's how she is, and I feel like the luckiest person around.

———— ✿ ————

NEW EXPERIENCES
Ellen Boldt

My youngest son was soon to get married, and I just wasn't feeling right. Noticing I had to urinate all the time, I had myself checked out and was told I had a reoccurring urinary tract infection. The doctor kept giving me antibiotics but the infection wasn't clearing up. Eventually, a biopsy determined I had a cancerous tumor in my bladder—unusual for a forty-six-year-old woman.

Years ago, they didn't have MRI or the testing we have today. A liver scan was done, and a lump was also discovered in the right quadrant of my abdomen. They knew then I had a non-cancerous cyst located around my liver and had to remove 80 percent of the liver. I stayed in the hospital for two weeks.

Six weeks later I had ostomy surgery. They felt positive they had stopped the bladder cancer by having the urostomy done on me. It was quite traumatic for me. I was more concerned with having to live with a bag on my abdomen than I worried about having cancer. Even though the doctor said the cancer was cured with the urostomy, the bag still bothered me.

My husband, Charles, and I were intimate; we had a very good sex life. The only thing I worried about with him was if the bag was going to be repugnant to him. He was extremely supportive as I lay in the hospital for another two weeks, weakened from the previous surgery I had dealing with the cyst.

I had an enterostomal therapist that was like an angel. She came in one day while my husband was there and said to me, "Tomorrow I am going to show you how to change the appliance."

My husband asked, "Could I come to watch?"

The thought of being intimate didn't bother him as much as it bothered me. I wondered how I was going to get through this awkward situation of wearing the bag.

At first I didn't want him to see the bag while we were having sex. I made my own little sex pants. They were pretty little lace panties, and I cut a slit in the crotch and that's what we did at first. Those pants helped me in the beginning and made me feel better about myself. Those lace panties weren't necessary for him. After a while, we tossed them aside.

We never discussed intimacy before the operation. We just thought this is another bump in the road. I had abdominal surgery before that with an appendectomy, a hysterectomy, and I guess I worked my way up, including gall bladder surgery. There was very little left to do, although I still had my tonsils. Just about everything else was removed.

We never thought it was going to be a problem. He was willing to change my appliance and he would help me. He would stick with me and guide me. The appliance wasn't a wafer like they are these days; it has separate pieces and a face plate that was a hard, green, rubber material. I had two and always had one ready. It was held in place by an O-ring. I had to put several parts together and hold them together with a rubber band. I was reluctant to switch to something different. I could not imagine not putting contact cement on my appliance anymore. I put a coat of it on the face plate and some around my stoma. I rolled about a four-by-four gauze bandage to keep the urine off the skin while I changed the appliance.

We did discuss the concern that I may have an accident. I always emptied my bag before those intimate moments so, in case it came off, there wouldn't be much urine. We decided we would take a shower together. I should have done that before I had a urostomy. Soon we started looking for excuses to take showers.

Charles hated it when I had to do something personal for him like changing a dressing, but he was always so supportive of me. Before he went to work in the morning, he came into the bathroom and helped me shower. He would put these fluffy white socks on me. He made sure I had something prepared for my lunch and then came home and fixed dinner too while I was recovering for those first couple of months.

I was a fussy housekeeper. When I got sick, he would clean the toilet, do the floor, even vacuumed. I learned that having a really clean house is not that important. I changed my priorities after urostomy surgery. I learned to live each day and have fun. I figured if my house was clean enough to be healthy, that's all we needed.

Accidents were a rare thing. It was only a couple of years after surgery when, once in a restaurant, I was drinking my fancy drink and suddenly I felt dampness. Thank goodness I was carrying around an extra set of products. I just said, "I have got to go." My husband and sister knew what was going on; they turned pale. I excused myself and changed my pouch in a restroom. They were standing outside the restroom nervously waiting for me. Our night was not ruined; I had done a good thing. I handled it.

When I first had these life-threatening experiences, I wondered, *why did this happen to me?* Now I know why. I have been able to help so many people along the way who felt desperate, and with a phone call or a visit, I know I have made a difference in their lives.

I had a grandson that passed away at age fourteen from cancer. I was angry that I was spared and my grandson didn't get to live. I have accepted it even though I still don't understand it. I do know that helping other people is what I am supposed to do.

I've been living with an ostomy almost forty years. I realize there are advantages at times. I don't need to stand outside a ladies room crossing my legs. I can say, "Go ahead of me, I can hold it." These days I line dance, do Tai Chi, stay active in our ostomy support group, and am president and editor of the newsletter. It's a good life.

———— ✆ ————

MIRACLES NEVER CEASE
Marsha Curnyn

I was having lunch in a restaurant in Honolulu with my friend Sharon when I suddenly felt wet. I looked down, couldn't see anything, but decided I better go the bathroom to check things out. Even though I have had an ileostomy for forty-three years, I am still not immune to accidents.

As soon as I arrived, I realized the bag had come loose and the contents were all over my panties and beginning to get on my pants. I didn't have my cell phone. I didn't have extra clothing, and I was in a quandary on what to do. I just kept staying in the stall and eventually it was long enough to concern my friend. A short while later, Sharon came to check on me, "Marsha, are you okay?"

"No, my bag has come loose and my clothes are all messed up."

"Well, take them off and pass them under the door," she said. Sharon kindly washed them out in the sink while I changed my pouch. We went back into the restaurant with me in my wet pants, enjoyed our lunch, and continued as if nothing out of the ordinary had just happened.

Forty-three years earlier, at age thirteen, I was diagnosed with hemorrhoids because of rectal bleeding, which really was ulcerative colitis. Two years later, I had an acute attack of ulcerative colitis and, again, it was misdiagnosed as stomach flu. I became ill so quickly that I was hospitalized. A proctoscope finally revealed my problem.

After a two-week hospital stay, I was in a dire situation—no one could find a vein and the dehydration had become critical. I stayed in that local hospital until my veins began to collapse. In desperation, my mom told the doctor, "We have to do something." I ended up going to a different hospital two hours away. And so my journey began via ambulance, Mom by my side and Pop following in his car.

I was sent to the Medical College of Virginia in Richmond. After I arrived at the medical center, a doctor in the ER found a vein for the IV fluids. It was crucial to keep the IV going, so my parents sat at my bedside all night ensuring the needle remained in place. The next morning, the only room available was in pediatrics, which resulted in a larger room reserved for long-term patients. Fortunately, it had bench-style seating that would become my mom's bed for the next five months.

Mom watched over me with incredible protectiveness day after long day. One night, a nurse came in to give me pills. They were huge and I had trouble swallowing them. The other nurses crushed them into applesauce, making it easier to get them down. This nurse was determined I was going to swallow those pills until Mom rose up from her bed in defense of her child.

Pop drove up every weekend to visit and would sometimes bring aunts who had volunteered to come up and give Mom a break for the weekend. This became the only private time my parents had during my hospital stay.

For the next three months, Mom watched her little girl go through painful tests, use the bathroom fifteen to twenty times a day, lose weight down to sixty-seven pounds, and gradually get weaker. The doctors wanted to do everything possible to prevent altering my body since I was so young, but a decision had to be made. The doctors told my parents I needed an operation or I would die. Even with an operation, it was possible I wouldn't make it off the table. If I survived, I would need psychiatric help to cope with the changes they would have made to save my life.

Of course, my parents agreed to the surgery. In the third month of my stay, I had surgery; I was only fifteen years old. From that point, I recalled asking Mom, "Why did they tie me down like an animal?"

She explained, "You were hallucinating and tried to pull out your IV and pull off your pouch."

I had been saved by a brilliant surgeon, and now faced a new normal with an ileostomy. Hospital staff was not equipped to tell me how to emotionally prepare for something so foreign. Ileostomy pouches back in the sixties were bulky, made of rubber that held odor, and were kept on with a special rubber cement that left me far from secure. The hospital sent in a female ostomate much older than me to visit. I noticed she was wearing a full skirt to hide the bag. I kept thinking about school and wondering if I would have to dress matronly like her. *Wasn't it going to be hard enough just facing everyone and not knowing what to say?* I loved the ocean and swimming. *How would I ever wear a swimsuit again?*

I had much recuperation time ahead of me. There was a very special doctor that proved to be our guardian angel. Dr. Bailey would accompany me to my tests and hold my hand while doctors did their exams and having him there made the earlier pain more bearable. As an intern, he was privy to the doctor's conversations in and out of my room. He shared with Mom one day that if the doctors saw Mom becoming depressed or in any way negatively impacting me, she would no longer be allowed to stay in my room. As a reminder to her, each time he'd pass by the door, Dr. Bailey would look at her and flash a fake smile.

I was grateful to be alive and out of pain for the first time. Two more months of hospitalization followed. There were many trials for Mom and me as I began the slow process of recuperating and regaining strength. I had to learn to care for my new stoma, which I affectionately named "Valerie (the volcano)." There were days of pouches breaking loose and horrible messes to clean up. Mom was there to help every step of the way. I realized later what a sacrifice it must have been to leave her home and husband and sleep in uncomfortable conditions, while being on constant guard.

Months later, Mom was at the local medical supply store one day buying supplies for me. She was informed there was a man who had left his name in case anyone needed a visitor or mentor to guide them through this difficult recovery with the ostomy. There was so much to learn about caring for the stoma and doctors were of little help. This seemed like an answer to a prayer, possibly.

Mom invited Hank Gilbert over for a visit. He came to our home wearing slacks without pleats; he was happy, vibrant, funny, and just what I needed.

"I deliberately wore this style of pants so you can see you can dress normally." Hank shared humorous stories of accidents he'd had with his pouch, and I learned he embraced those horrible moments with humor and resilience. It gave me hope and peace of mind. Mom was thrilled that she'd taken the chance to reach out to this man and life took a dramatic positive turn that day.

About thirty years later, I was in a medical supply store while visiting my sister. Living halfway around the world, I wasn't expecting to see anyone I knew. While being helped, a man came in and waited for his turn. We glanced at each other, and then looked again. *Could it be?* I asked him a couple of questions and soon realized I was reunited with my angel from many years ago.

Hank recognized me too, and we embraced like two long lost friends. We caught up on each other's lives and he asked if my parents still lived in the home he'd visited so many years ago. I told Hank about my mom's own poor health. She'd had breast cancer and a radical mastectomy at age thirty-three, followed by many other health challenges. She lived to see me go back to high school, get dressed up for proms, attend college, get married, and begin a normal, healthy life of my own. At age sixty-four, she succumbed to lung cancer knowing that I was okay. Seeing Hank again made me appreciate all the love and care I was given, especially by my mother.

Today I am fifty-eight years old and have had a full and active life. I am married, and have enjoyed skiing, white-water rafting, hiking, traveling to foreign countries, and still love the ocean. My clothes have never shown any hint that my body is altered. I have learned what a difference other people have made in my life, and I hope I can do the same for others. Miracles continue to be a part of my life.

———— ⊛ ————

GET OUT OF YOUR COMFORT ZONE
Patti Iverson

Here's the secret to a long and healthy marriage. It's not saying I love you or I am sorry, it's being able to let it go. That's the only way to get along with a mother-in-law. We've been married forty years through my husband having multiple sclerosis and a heart attack, plus me with my asthma and diabetes. We must be real diehards—crazy—or just still in love after all these years together. We've cared for my husband's dad dealing with Alzheimer's, and Randy's ninety-five-year-old mom still lives with us after twenty-five years. Randy was a fire chief for thirty-five years, and I am a clown and Mrs. Claus.

Despite what we've been through, the pouch was an adjustment, but I soon realized I was stupid to suffer for so long fighting the bag. My lover and hunk of a husband turned into my caregiver. My hands shook like the proverbial bowlful of jelly. My tummy wouldn't hold food. My heart was not in the right place for loving, and as for my new stoma—fergeddaboudit! Effluent oozed out 24/7 all around the stoma, not properly out of one hole.

Randy would be kneeling at my feet, which most women would adore, 'cept I was sitting on the toilet wailing pitifully. He'd go through emptying my pouch and then I vomited all over his back. Oh, gross.

Sex was another story altogether. We've successfully and physically loved through pregnancies, hysterectomies, surgeries galore on both of us, broken bones, periods, mothers-in-law in the next room, all the stuff of life—trials and joys. But an ileostomy—a bag of poop on my stomach—threw me for a loop.

But soon it became apparent that wasn't what was on Randy's mind in any way, shape, or fashion once we got into showing love to each other. He had his mind on other things. Then I knew I was going be an okay wife and lover and, with acceptance, came joy.

Just hang in there and get out of your comfort zone into your sexy zone. If I get out of myself and concentrate more on him, then bingo, it's better for both of us.

———— ✿ ————

ANIMAL CAREGIVERS
DIANNA HOPPE

Sometimes it feels like life is crashing down around you. After moving my mother here to Illinois from Texas and tending to her, she died from renal failure. I had already lost my brother and father, and I was starting to fall ill myself with diverticulitis, thinking I was getting an ulcer. Constipation had always been a struggle, too, that left me with a sick feeling. After Mom died, I was devastated when Joe, my significant other of twenty-five years, was diagnosed with cancer. I cared for him for two years before he died. Just two weeks later, I was rushed to the hospital for an emergency colostomy.

It was a vulnerable time for me; I was physically and emotionally weak with no one to greet me, to help me, to look after me. My friends were a disappointment; they were nowhere to be found. A cab driver brought me home from the hospital and made sure I got into my house safely.

When I walked into my home, my spirits were lifted temporarily because my animals were there to greet me. It became obvious soon enough that my house was in disarray and my animals had been neglected. Sadly, Sabrina my cat who had a thyroid condition, died two weeks after my return. I also have a cat named OK, short for Oklahoma. I was driving from Chicago to Dallas to see my mother and brother one Christmas many years ago. On the turnpike south of Tulsa, there was a family of kittens swished off the side of the road, except for the little guy, who was just sitting there with his eyes all aglow. I had to stop; he's thirteen years old now and still happy.

Although the animals could not tend to me, I knew they were there for me. They would lie with me and in their own special way try to heal me, motivate me, and give me their strength and support. When I truly needed someone—something to help pull me through, it was the creatures that did it. They do miraculous things for others and in their own way, they cared for me. They gave me a reason to get up in the morning, even if it was only to tend to their needs and perhaps only pet their little faces and feed them. They gave me the sense of enjoyment and pleasure, while asking so little from me.

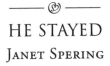

HE STAYED
Janet Spering

Facebook is a great way to hook up with old friends. I am dating Dave, someone I originally met when I was fourteen and he was sixteen. I looked him up last year and we've been together since. I told him at our first meeting at Starbucks that I didn't look sick, but I had just gone through cancer. A suspicious polyp in a routine colonoscopy led to a diagnosis of rectal cancer. At age fifty-three, I had no symptoms. Chemo and radiation became part of my life, along with surgery for an ostomy. He didn't seem fazed by it, but I don't think he really understood it for a couple of months.

I was feeling very sick, and I asked Dave if he would walk the dog. "Absolutely—sure," and he came right over to take the dog out.

While he was gone I had really bad diarrhea in the bag. When I removed my bag, it shot out all over the bathroom like a volcano. I was in shock and just stood there watching it.

He came back into the condo and said, "I think somehow I got dog pooh on my shoe."

I had put on a bag and crawled into bed. I was too sick to clean up the mess left behind.

"Don't go into the bathroom," I warned.

He ignored me and that is when he realized how sick I was. There were feces all over the wall and the floor and splashed up on the surfaces. I didn't know that projectile poop was possible. Of course, I was incredibly embarrassed; I am the kind of person that likes to take care of things myself.

Dave just went in to clean it up, he was whistling and singing and cleaned it up as he talked about his three kids, "The stuff I've had to clean up with them with their pooping and throwing up incidents, you wouldn't believe."

He made me feel comforted and like it was no big deal. He kept coming in to check up on me, I was still green and shaking. Dave told me to relax and asked if I needed water or anything. Then he asked, "Do you want me to spend the night to keep an eye on you?"

I hadn't slept with him and he still cleaned up my poop.

The first time we were intimate, I had a wrap around my ostomy, but Dave didn't care so I didn't cover it. I explained to him that there is no muscle control and things can come out at will and at the most inappropriate times. When I showed him my stoma, that is when the poop decided to come out. I put on a fresh one before going to bed. I have had other blow outs after surgery, but as he said, he could not conceive leaving someone when they are that sick. A lot of guys might have run the other way, but not Dave.

—— ✿ ——

TIP THE WAITER
Kathi T. and Steven D.

When my wife first had her ileostomy, we would find ourselves trying to discuss it in public without it being embarrassing to her, or uncomfortable for people who might overhear us. She had been having so many troubles that she would have to go to the bathroom to check her bag twice an hour, no matter where we were.

I suggested we use a secret code so she could feel more comfortable discussing it in public. We decided that the code would be "tip the waiter."

It was only a few days later when we went to dinner at a local Cheesecake Factory, when my wife suddenly got up very quickly from the table.

I asked, "Where are you going?"

She said, "I have to go 'tip the waiter.'"

Being a typical guy with a short memory, I asked, "Can't I just put it on my Visa?"

You should have seen the smile on her face, and the confusion on mine.

It was the first time we laughed about something she had felt was such an unfunny situation.

——— ✿ ———

THE LIGHT IS GETTING BRIGHTER
ROSALIND SAVAGE

When I read that Brenda was doing this book, for some inexplicable reason, I contacted her to tell my story. We had the most wonderful conversation; she was extremely inspiring. You see, I have never spoken to a person with an ostomy in all of my twenty-six-plus years of having an ileostomy. She was motivational, and I have begun looking at my situation differently. I liken it to starting on my second life, trying to be bitter-free. I am walking through a dark tunnel with a lantern, but the light gets brighter and brighter as I travel.

I wonder what kind of man I would have had if I didn't have an ostomy. With the men I've dealt with, you get to a point when you have to tell them you wear a pouch. I have never met anyone who was not understanding and kind. They weren't acting. Men were drawn to me in a flirtatious, normal way. After several dates, I would lead up to the conversation about the pouch, something like a doctor talking to a patient. "This is what I have because I had to have my colon removed."

I remember one man saying that it is not what you wear, or what your illness is, it's the kind of person you are. He told me about his father and that both of his legs were off and how he got around in a wheelchair and was more of a man than most. Most of the time there was no response. I never asked them how they felt about it. Many of them went through my illness because they had to deal with me being in the hospital and it just became a normal pattern. That became my life and that is who I was.

The operation changed my life forever. It was debilitating for me physically and emotionally. I had grown very bitter about it. There was no way I could find the humor in it. I was suffering daily because I was dehydrated and had problems with leaking. I was going through three to four pouches a day. At this point in life, age fifty-eight, with all I was going through, I wasn't interested in dealing with men.

I've always believed there was a reason for everything, but I had a tough time discovering the reason for this one. It hasn't been revealed—yet. Maybe it is to help people deal with life as an ostomate but I haven't gotten there quite yet; I still fight off too much bitterness. The last time I was with someone was quite some time ago. We were engaged to be married. I had an accident one night while we were in bed, the pouch had opened up, and he jumped out of bed indignantly saying, "All your s—t's on me." I cleaned up and felt dirty and ashamed; he slept elsewhere. I don't know what he expected. His behavior shocked me into a trauma of sorts. I had read someplace we could have made a joke out of it, that seemed impossible. I never did get over it.

It's been ten years and since then I haven't wanted to deal with anybody. When I was younger, I could deal with having the conversation. I can't do that now. That experience was too demoralizing.

It was at that point when Brenda who had been listening and not saying anything broke in to express a need to say something. She apologized for expressing her opinion because she's tried to keep each interview objective, but she admitted she could no longer stay silent as I told my story.

Until I talked to Brenda, I had assumed responsibility for his actions and in a way took blame for the accident. She made me see this was in fact his problem, which he couldn't see past his own crap. I had sat in that shame and relived that awkward situation for years, not allowing myself to know another man or put myself in a position to even talk to a man where it might lead to the fact that I would have to tell them I had an ostomy. I had removed myself from any possibilities of that happening and, essentially, I severed my sexuality and wouldn't allow myself to be put in a position of ever expressing it again.

There have been men that were interested in me, but I would only go so far into the friendship before I curtailed it. I also couldn't imagine going to a support group where I might laugh about it; I couldn't fathom that; I didn't feel brave at all.

Things have improved for me and the journey continues. As I travel, I am less bitter and more positive. This happened when I finally accepted the fact that circumstances were not going to change, and then I opened my eyes to see that I have lived a very blessed life. As my mother says, "Tomorrow is not promised to any of us." Therefore, why waste any more of my precious time and needless energy being bitter about something I cannot change. The key is to seek help when needed and be open to endless possibilities in the future. That light keeps getting brighter.

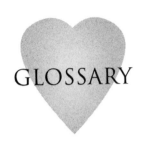

GLOSSARY

– A –

Appliance: another term for ostomy pouch.

– B –

B-cell non-Hodgkin Lymphoma: cancer that originates in your lymphatic system, the disease-fighting network spread throughout your body.

– C –

C-diff (Clostridium Difficile): a bacterium that can cause symptoms ranging from diarrhea to life-threatening inflammation of the colon.

Colectomy: surgery during which all or part of the colon is removed.

Colostomy: a surgical operation that creates an opening from the colon to the surface of the body to function as an anus.

Conseal plug: a lubricated foam plug that is attached to an adhesive ring and expands in the stoma like a tampon. Prevents feces from leaving the bowel and has a filter to allow gas to expel.

Crohn's disease: an inflammatory disease of the intestines that may affect any part of the gastrointestinal tract from mouth to anus, causing a wide variety of symptoms.

CT scan or CAT: Computerized Axial Tomography.

Cystoscope: a thin-lighted tube inserted into the urethra for testing.

– D –

Diverticulitis: swelling or inflammation of an abnormal pouch in the intestinal wall.

– E –

ED: erectile dysfunction.

eHarmony: an online dating website that matches men and women with other singles.

– F –

FAP: Familial Adenomatous Polyposis, an inherited colorectal cancer syndrome.

Fistulas: an abnormal connection or passageway between two epithelium-lined organs or vessels that normally do not connect.

Fobbed: to cheat or deceive.

– G –

Gardner Syndrome: also known as familial colorectal polyposis (multiple polyps in the colon together with tumors outside of the colon).

– I –

IBD: Inflammatory Bowel Disease.

IBS: Irritable Bowel Syndrome.

ICU: Intensive Care Unit.

Ileostomy: surgical procedure that creates an opening from the ileum through the abdominal wall to function as an anus.

Ileal Conduit: urinary diversion.

Impacted bowels: when feces become trapped in the lower part of the large intestine, causing a waste obstruction.

– J –

J-pouch: an internal pouch to hold stool that is created from the last part of the small intestine and attached to the anus or the remainder of the rectum.

– K –

Knee trembler: making love to the point the knees tremble.

Koch pouch: a continent ileostomy for stool or urine, the patient inserts a catheter to empty the pouch.

– L –

Laparoscopically: a modern surgical technique in which operations in the abdomen are performed through small incisions.

Loo: toilet.

– M –

Match.com: online dating site and resource for personals and singles.

MeetAnOstoMate.com: will help you get in touch with ostomates in your area and around the world.

– N –

Nappies: diapers.

– O –

Ostomate: a person who has had an ostomy, which is a surgical operation to create an opening in the body for the discharge of body wastes.

– P –

Panproctocolectomy: the surgical removal of the whole rectum and the colon.

Peritonitis: inflammation of the peritoneum.

Pratt: idiot.

Proctitis: inflammation of the rectum, marked by bloody stools and a frequent urge to defecate.

PTSD: post-traumatic stress disorder.

– Q –

Queue: line.

– S –

Short bowel syndrome: a malabsorption disorder caused by the surgical removal of the small intestine.

Sod off: get lost.

– T –

TPN: Total Parenteral Nutrition.

– U –

Ulcerative colitis: a serious chronic inflammatory disease of the large intestine and rectum characterized by recurrent episodes of abdominal pain, fever, chills, and profuse diarrhea.

UOAA: United Ostomy Associations of America.

Ureter: thick-walled tubes that carry urine from the kidney to the urinary bladder.

Urostomy: a stoma for the urinary system; made in cases where long-term drainage of urine through the bladder and urethra is not possible.

– W –

WOCN: Wound Ostomy Continence Nurse.

INTIMATE WEAR, POUCH COVERS, AND OSTOMY RESOURCES

Bag It, www.bagit.biz, 763-434-3175

Better Life Ostomy Belt, www.ostomysolutions.com, 661-575-9240

C&M Ostomy Supplies, www.cmostomysupply.com, 954-234-7120

Intimate Wear, www.intimatemomentsapparel.com, 201-825-9486

Kangaroo Medical Products, www.kmedpro.com, 417-831-1564

My Coveralls, www.mycoveralls.com, 304-724-7286

My Heart Ties, www.myheartties.com, 888-338-TIES

Options, www.options-ostomy.com, 800-736-6555

Ostaway x-Bag, www.bagitaway.com, 800-774-6097

Ostomy Secrets, www.ostomysecrets.com, 877-613-6246

Pouch Pals, www.pouchpals.com, 618-537-4329

Sto Med, www.sto-med.com, 800-814-4195

The Celebration Inc., www.celebrationostomysupportbelt.com, 413-539-7704

Vanilla Blush, www.vblush.com, Europe # +44 14176 30991

Weir Comfees Ostomy Wear, www.weircomfees.com, 866-856-5088

White Rose Collection, www.whiterosecollection.com, UK # (0)1202-854634

Yentl's Secret's, www.yentlssecrets.com, 800-749-3685

United Ostomy Association of America, Inc., www.uoaa.org, 800-826-0826

WOCN (Wound Ostomy Continence Nurses Society), www.wocn.org, 888-224-9626

CCFA (Crohn's & Colitis Foundation of America), www.ccfa.org, 800-932-2423

C3 life Online Ostomy Community, www.C3Life.com

Online Ostomy Community, www.MeetAnOstoMate.com

Coloplast, www.coloplast.com, 888-726-7872

Convatec, www.Convatec.com, 800-422-8811

Cymed, www.cymedostomy.com, 800-582-0707

Kem Enterprises Osto-EZ-Ven, www.kemonline.com, 888-562-8802

Hollister, www.hollister.com, 888-740-8999

Marlen, www.marlenmfg.com, 216-292-7060

Nu Hope, www.nu-hope.com, 800-899-5017

Brenda Elsagher, www.livingandlaughing.com

CONTRIBUTOR BIOGRAPHIES

Alistair of Scotland—I enjoy fishing, the outdoors, wildlife, and anything that moves, but my real passion is traveling and eating local foods, especially Italy. ajr@totalise.co.uk

Carla Anderson—Carla and Anthony live in California, love spending time with their two daughters, and enjoy playing darts. Recently Anthony had miraculous surgery and is healing faster each day and they feel hope again. carla.anderson@live.com

Big Trev (Anonymous)—Big Trev lives alone in a lovely one bedroom apartment situated in a beautiful suburban area of Belfast in Northern Ireland. He continues to enjoy a few drinks now and then, travels quite a bit, and tries to live life to the full. musitrev@gmail.com

Louise (Anonymous)—Louise is fifty-eight, lives in Atlanta, GA, enjoys reading, doing creative coloring, listening to jazz, watching a good western, and loves her four children. Her favorite saying is, "Let every action, reaction, thought, and emotion be based on love." dallce2@yahoo.com

Matt (Anonymous)—Matt, forty, lives in Baltimore, MD, working in health care policy on the state level and in Washington, D.C. and has had an ileostomy due to ulcerative colitis since age eighteen and is proud of having one of the first straight pull-throughs done that failed. He enjoys playing blues and rock on the electric guitar, hiking, working out, and spending time with his wife and two dogs. M_L_M_1950@yahoo.com

Michael R. (Anonymous)—Michael lives in Minnesota, works in television, enjoys golfing, hiking, and dating. He appreciates his twelve-step program, and feeling physically fit. alohamike@hotmail.com

Morgan (Anonymous)—Sometimes life throws you a curve. You think your problems are solved with surgery, and suddenly you're back in the dating pool—or shark tank. It doesn't have to be scary; being single after ostomy surgery in my twenties wasn't always what it was cracked up to be but sometimes it did crack me up.

Steven D. and Kathi T. (Anonymous)—Steven and Kathi hail from Arlington, MA. Kathi has had an ileostomy for three years after a near fatal bout of toxic megacolon.

Sue (Anonymous)—While trying to be fit and keep those aches and pains at bay by exercising three days a week, Sue stays involved with her ostomy group. For relaxation, she likes watercolor painting and reading, even while traveling to far off lands. SAHR786@msn.com

Andrew and Vanessa Baker—Vanessa enjoys nature and photography while Andrew's passion is putting Vanessa's photos on the computer. They live in Abbeyleix, Ireland, with three dogs, and their lads are grown now—one lives in Australia and the other in Kilkenny. abdl9@eircom.net

Bob Baker—Bob Baker lived with ulcerative colitis for twenty-seven years and at age forty was diagnosed with stage II colon cancer and now lives with a permanent ileostomy. He says he loves his ostomy for giving him his health back and enjoys spending life with his wife and three children in Connecticut. bobbaker@uoaa.org

Maria Barker—Since telling my story, our son got married, my ex-husband asked me back, and I told him where to go. I have met a new man and my life is a lot richer because I thank God for making me the way I am—I'll be grateful if my story helps anyone. barkermaria98@yahoo.com

Dawn Becker—Dawn is a mom to four kids, a business owner who loves the arts, and she's expanding her businesses to include a Paint Your Own Pottery and a Gourmet Marshmallow company. Her favorite motto is, "Never regret anything that made you smile." dbecker119@yahoo.com

Pam Bennett—Pam likes photography for use in cards and books for her family. She is a keen member of her local fishing club and enjoys watching rugby with a glass of lager. pamandraybennett@talktalk.net

Sarah Biggart—Sarah grew up in San Diego, CA, where she lives in and runs a group home for developmentally disabled adults. She is happily married to husband, Jason, and mother to son, Hendrix, and enjoys photography, volunteering, and practicing kung fu.

Ellen Boldt—Ellen lives in Florida and is president and editor of the newsletter for the Hernando County Ostomy Association and enjoys visits with her growing family. In her spare time she does tai chi, line dancing, and loves to read. ellenboldt@att.net

Nancy and Gary Chow—Nancy and Gary Chow live in San Francisco, CA. Having both lost their previous spouses to cancer, Nancy is utilizing her experiences as an ileostomate and a WOC Nurse to help others dealing with similar issues, and Gary manages patient service programs as a Community Mission Director for the American Cancer Society.

Cheryl Cleveland—Cheryl lives in Tennessee with her son, Noah, and husband, Bert. They like to go camping and spend family time together playing board games and outside activities. crc865@yahoo.com

Marsha Curnyn—Marsha Curnyn is a happily married, retired editor with the federal government residing in Alexandria, VA. She is also an eight-year survivor of bladder cancer. thecurnyns@gmail.com

Cherie DeGroot—Cherie and Skip live in Green Bay, WI. Cherie's motto is "Never take life for granted and never give up hope." UGogrl51@aol.com

Liz Dennis—Diagnosed with stage III rectal cancer at age thirty-nine in May 2006, in Tempe, AZ, I had a temporary ileostomy for a year, ending up with a permanent colostomy. My passion is advocating for awareness of colorectal cancer, and I've lobbied congress on a national level and run a local support group for colorectal patients. 66Rose@q.com

Andy Fletcher—Andy lives on the South Coast in the UK, and is married with a stepdaughter. He enjoys foreign holidays in the Mediterranean where he and Julie hope to one day retire. His diary of the operation is at www.mystoma.co.uk.

Leslie Gilbert-Grunder—Leslie is currently writing books for children and is glad she doesn't have to take so many bathroom breaks anymore. leslie-g@hotmail.com

Steven Goldberg—Steven Goldberg remains active in the school counseling profession and lives a life full of love, passion, and laughter. He is passionate about his family and is a fierce advocate for people with digestive disorders. incrediberg@gmail.com

Esten Gose—Esten enjoys playing sports, snowboarding, and hanging out with friends. He is active in the UOAA, and is chairperson of YODAA and on the UOAA ASG Advisory Board. gose.esten@gmail.com

Aileen Gould—Licensed Mental Health Counselor, resides in Glen Cove, New York and enjoys working with people throughout the United States with chronic illnesses via the telephone. She enjoys nature, music, and helping others heal. 1soulful@optonline.net

Teresa Guzman—Teresa, twenty-six, was diagnosed with peri-anal Crohn's disease in January 2007, and had her colon and rectum removed February 2010. She recently graduated from the Thomas M. Cooley Law School and lives with her husband, their Doberman, their rabbit, their bird, and their fish in West Michigan.

Michael Hassett—Michael lives in Long Island, NY, runs two ostomy meetings monthly, is grateful for the freedom and the new family the ostomy brought into his life, and is delighted to help others in their journey. He enjoys the beach, saltwater, and time with his kids. atygla@aim.com

Cricket Henley—Cricket Henley is the director of communications for Ostomy Secrets. She and her husband, John, of twenty-six years, have two children. cricket@ostomysecrets.com

Dianna Hoppe—Dianna is a woman who keeps on keeping on and staying busy with a small business called *As the Tail Tells*. Dianna loves people, animals, plants, and things. stilldianna@att.net

Patti Iverson—Patti Iverson loves her Lord and her ministries to women, which include fancy schmancy tea parties and mentoring young mamas. She fills in time as the chief homemaker, being on the local board for child evangelism, and writing a column for *The Christian Journal* out of Medford, OR. randpi2@charter.net

Carland Kerr—Carland is known as the funny blonde who lives by the sea shore and loves to make jewelry. She and her husband love to travel, ride their Harley, and enjoy their two portly cats.

Barbara Kupferberg—Barbara Kupferberg has had an ileostomy for two years due to ulcerative colitis. She is an avid bridge player and enjoys time in Illinois and Florida and loves the fact that having her ileostomy allows her to travel around the world. babakup7@gmail.com

Carol Larson—Carol Larson was diagnosed with stage III colorectal cancer in 1999. Since then she has been co-president of the Ostomy Association of the Minneapolis Area (OAMA), awarded the 2008 "Breaking Boundaries Award" from fightcolorectalcancer.org, and has written two guidebooks to cope with colorectal cancer., *When The Trip Changes*, and *Positive Options for Colorectal Cancer.*

Donna Lemison—Donna is an air force veteran who lives in Florida, enjoys working with stained glass, the elderly at the nursing home, and volunteers at the Elks Club. She loves her three children, five grandchildren, and her dog. dlemison@att.net

Georga A. Linkous-Long—Georga lives in South Carolina, is a freelance salesperson for E K Designs Jewelry, and is a consultant and coach with her company, www.myostomateplace.com. ostomateplace@bellsouth.net

Kelly Livingston—Kelly lives in Utah, enjoys most sports, being outdoors, and appreciates life more each day. She loves foods of all types, despite being told with an ileostomy, she should restrict intake of certain food groups. nya065@gmail.com

David and Ceil McGee—David and Ceil live in Charlotte, NC, and are active in their United Methodist Church. They have a white fur ball of a dog named Wally and an appropriately named/colored kitty, Punkin. David-Ceil.McGee@Inbox.com

Veralynne Malone—Veralynne is a fifty-five-year ostomate who is married to the most wonderful man in the world. They have three wonderful children and two grandchildren with another on the way. Veralynne works and is very happy with life, ostomy and all.

Gordon Maney—Gordon Maney is a mechanic, writer, teacher, forester, and student of life. He lives among the trees in rural Iowa County, IA.

Doug Marchant—Doug is a veteran of the ostomy life who admits to learning something new every day. He enjoys fixing things and tinkering with tools, teaching his boys along the way, and enjoying the simple things in life with his wife, kids, and grandkids, especially cooking for them all. dug127@live.com

Lisa Mayfield—Lisa has spent more than half her life with an ostomy and because of that surgery she could work, carry, and raise her son, travel, coach, and meet wonderful people. She wouldn't choose it but at this point she wouldn't trade it either—it made her stronger, healthier, and more understanding. lilbitmo@bellsouth.net

Doug Milgram—Doug, a retired transportation engineer, lives with first wife in Elkview, WV, and spends as much time possible with his grandkids hunting and fishing. Doug spent almost forty years as a volunteer firefighter, first-aid squad member, and has recently been appointed to the ASG Advisory Board of the UOAA, something of which he is extremely proud. douginwv@gmail.com

Sari Mogol Legge—Sari does life coaching for IBD and ostomates (www.mogolmedianetcasting.net) and resides in Rhode Island with Peter and Jacob.

Nancy Olesky—Nancy lives in a suburb of Chicago, loves to read mysteries, go for walks, and cook. nanook60@sbcglobal.net

Jon O'Neill—After working in fourteen countries, Jon settled in Spain for sun, sea, sex, and sangria with wife, Joan. Interests are in diving, walking, traveling, dancing, reading, and integrating with the Spanish. jon@mazarronmail.com

Rosana Paz—I learned I have just this one life to live, and I want to enjoy all its colors deeply. It's never too late to start, having done it many times already—I'll never stop. rosanalic93@hotmail.com

George Salamy—George is a retired manager from AT&T and has traveled the world extensively having an ostomy for thirty-five years. After being widowed, he married Linda and now has five daughters and eight grandchildren. gfsalamy@comcast.net

Rosalind Savage—Rosalind Savage resides in Harlem, NY. She is a professional librarian and an expert in African American studies. At times she acts as a consultant on various library projects.

Fred Shulak—Fred is a retired professional and has many interests: cooking, music, piano, philosophy, religion, movies, antiques, and knitting. Formerly an officer of his ostomy chapter, in 2005, he became the co-chairperson of the GLO network and has served as its sole chairperson since 2006. thadbear773@yahoo.com

Christina Sowell—Christina Sowell continues to flourish in life with IBD in the all-encompassing roles of daughter, wife, mother, grandmother, artist, IBD support group director, and participant. Blessed with love and relentless support of a strong and caring family, Christina feels a greater sense of confidence and self-esteem to manage the hurdles of life with IBD. csowell21@comcast.net

Janet Spering—I have an ostomy, but it doesn't define me. I'm a woman, sister, cousin, friend, and daughter, who loves photography, my dogs, Dave, Cape Cod, Paris, Japan, hiking, biking, traveling, and life.

Holly St. Jean—Holly St. Jean is an English teacher at a regional high school in central Massachusetts. Her personal essay "The Two-Step" appears in an anthology entitled *Queer Girls in Class*. hmsj1223@msn.com

Anita and William Summers—William and Anita are retired and live in Tucson, AZ. They enjoy visiting their children and grandchildren, making jewelry, watching their favorite TV shows, and walking in the outdoors. Meilandra@gmail.com

Cindy Sylvia—Cindy Sylvia is a Certified Wound Ostomy and Continence Nurse who happens to love life as a person with an ileostomy. Always open to new experiences, she has recently become an entrepreneur, opening her own business in fine intimate (www.mycoveralls.com) wear for ostomy pouches.

Charlotte Taylor—Charlotte lives in Alabama and Missouri, has two grown sons, Jerry and Jeff, and a grandson and granddaughter. She loves sewing, quilting, going for walks, and bowling. noodles5642@gmail.com

Marcella Taylor-Billing—I do Aquafit three to four times a week for exercise, like gardening, reading, and cooking for others. I am known as the London Boat lady by some and am glad to have a stoma so I can live life to the fullest. redrumian@yahoo.co.uk

Judy Tipton—Judy and Carrol live in the smoky mountains of Tennessee and love spending time with their two wonderful daughters, their helpful stepson, and five grandsons. They enjoy attending church together, gardening, and helping the elderly.

Patrick Tobin—Pat dealt with the effects of UC for twenty years and has had an ileostomy since 2007. He lives in the Memphis area and enjoys wood-working, biking, and backpacking and in the summer of 2009, he spent five days hiking on a section of the Appalachian Trail with his son and a group of boy scouts.

Dave Uri—Dave is thirty-three, lives in Minnesota, enjoys the WAC (We are Crohn's) group on Facebook, YODAA, and has participated in the GYGIG bike ride. Currently studying Japanese, he also enjoys cooking, watching movies, going on dates, and his cat named Luna. dave.uri@gmail.com

Dawn Vander Haar—Dawn lives in South Dakota, loves to read and hang out with family. She is a grandmother to four wonderful grandkids and has lived with an ostomy for six years.

Lisa Waldron—Lisa lives in El Paso, TX, with her husband, son, baby on the way, and two dogs. She loves spending time with her family, hiking, weight lifting, and mountain biking.

ABOUT THE AUTHOR

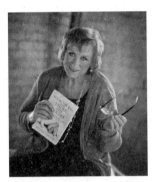

B renda Elsagher is an international speaker, author, and comic. She and her family live in Burnsville, Minnesota. This is her fourth book and when she is not writing or speaking, she enjoys traveling, playing scrabble, riding her bike, watching movies, reading, and visiting with friends.

You can read Brenda's humorous columns in the Secure Start Newsletter by Hollister Incorporated that comes out quarterly. Enroll at www.Hollister.com or call 1-888-740-8999 to receive your complimentary issue today.

Brenda also writes a weekly journal blog for www.C3life.com.

Looking for a funny, poignant speaker for your next event? Brenda would love to come to your area to speak for your organization, please call her at 952-882-9882 or e-mail: Brenda@livingandlaughing.com. Brenda's website: www.livingandlaughing.com.